**rses**

## Second Edition

Philip Jevon
RGN, BSc (Hon), PGCE, ENB 124
Resuscitation Officer/Clinical Skills Lead
Honorary Clinical Lecturer
Manor Hospital
Walsall
UK

*Consulting Editor*
Jawad M. Khan
BioMed Sci (Hons), MBBS, MRCP (Lon)
Consultant Interventional Cardiologist and
Honorary Senior Lecturer
City Hospital, Birmingham
UK

⟨W⟩ **WILEY-BLACKWELL**

A John Wiley & Sons, Ltd., Publication

This edition first published 2009
© first edition published 2003
This edition © 2009 by Philip Jevon
© 2003 by Blackwell Publishing Ltd

Blackwell Publishing was acquired by John Wiley & Sons in February 2007.
Blackwell's publishing programme has been merged with Wiley's global
Scientific, Technical, and Medical business to form Wiley-Blackwell.

Registered office
John Wiley & Sons Ltd, The Atrium, Southern Gate, Chichester, West
Sussex, PO19 8SQ, United Kingdom

Editorial Offices
2121 State Avenue, Ames, Iowa 50014-8300, USA
9600 Garsington Road, Oxford, OX4 2DQ, United Kingdom

For details of our global editorial offices, for customer services and for
information about how to apply for permission to reuse the copyright
material in this book please see our website at www.wiley.com/
wiley-blackwell.

The right of the author to be identified as the author of this work has been
asserted in accordance with the Copyright, Designs and Patents Act 1988.

Library of Congress Cataloging-in-Publication Data

Jevon, Philip.
ECGs for nurses / Phillip Jevon. – 2nd ed.
p. ; cm. – (Essential clinical skills for nurses)
Includes bibliographical references and index.
ISBN 978-1-4051-8162-4 (pbk. : alk. paper)  1. Electrocardiography.
2. Arrhythmia–Nursing.  I. Title.  II. Series: Essential clinical skills
for nurses.
[DNLM: 1. Electrocardiography–Nurses' Instruction.  2. Arrhythmias,
Cardiac–prevention & control–Nurses' Instruction.  WG 140 J58e 2009]
RC683.5.E5J48 2009
616.1′207547–dc22
2009009895

A catalogue record for this book is available from the British Library.

Set in 9 on 11 pt Palatino by SNP Best-set Typesetter Ltd., Hong Kong
Printed and bound in Malaysia by KHL Printing Co Sdn Bhd

1   2009

# Contents

*Foreword* iv
*Acknowledgements* vi

Chapter 1    The conduction system in the heart    1

Chapter 2    Principles of ECG monitoring    10

Chapter 3    ECG interpretation of cardiac arrhythmias    40

Chapter 4    Cardiac arrhythmias originating in the SA node    50

Chapter 5    Cardiac arrhythmias originating in the atria    72

Chapter 6    Cardiac arrhythmias originating in the AV junction    96

Chapter 7    Cardiac arrhythmias originating in the ventricles    114

Chapter 8    Cardiac arrhythmias with atrioventricular block    135

Chapter 9    Cardiac arrhythmias associated with cardiac arrest    155

Chapter 10    Recording a 12 lead ECG    169

Chapter 11    Interpreting a 12 lead ECG    182

Chapter 12    Management of peri-arrest arrhythmias    220

Chapter 13    Record keeping    243

*Appendix* 249
*Index* 286

# Foreword

I am absolutely delighted to write the foreword for the second edition of *ECGs for Nurses* on request of the author Phil Jevon. Phil has vast experience in emergency and cardiac care and has published widely, especially in the field of resuscitation, monitoring the critically ill patient and ECGs for nurses.

'Diseases of the heart and circulatory system are the main cause of death in the UK and account for almost 198,000 deaths each year' (British Heart Foundation, 2008, p. 12).

'Cardiac arrhythmias affects more than 700,000 people in England and is consistently in the top ten reasons for hospital admission' (Department of Health, 2005, p. 3).

'Delivering improved quality of initial and early care for patients with arrhythmia will lead to these cases being managed more quickly, more cost effectively and in appropriate settings with improved quality of life and survival outcomes' (Department of Health, 2005, p. 3). For this to happen, however, nurses must have the skills to recognise arrhythmia and know how to manage them; this is where *ECGs for Nurses* can be very helpful.

*ECGs for Nurses* explores arrhythmia analysis as well as 12 lead ECG recording, which are both crucial skills for nurses looking after patients with cardiovascular disease and or arrhythmias.

The systematic approach to the whole book makes it very easy to follow and the logical progression in each chapter, which includes introduction, learning outcomes, systematic analysis of arrhythmia and 12 leads, with examples, signs and symptoms, and management, really helps with the application of knowledge and skills. The reference list at the end of each chapter encourages further reading and exploration.

I have enjoyed reading the second edition of this very useful ECG book and I hope that you will find it as useful and that it will enhance the care that you give to patients and their families.

*Cynthia Curtis*
*Head or Nurse Education & Events*
*British Heart Foundation,*
*Greater London House,*
*180 Hampstead Rd,*
*London.*
*NW1 7AW*

## REFERENCES

British Heart Foundation (2008) *Coronary Heart Disease Statistics 2008.* British Heart Foundation, London.

Department of Health (2005) Arrhythmias and sudden cardiac death. Chapter 8 in *Coronary Heart Disease.* Department of Health, London

# Acknowledgements

I am grateful to Dr Jawad M. Khan for meticulously checking the manuscript and ECG traces.

I am grateful to Cynthia Curtis for writing the foreword. Cynthia was the course leader for the ENB 124 Course which I attended at Newcastle RVI in 1988.

I am grateful to Steve Webb and Shareen Juwle for their help with some of the images.

I am grateful to staff on CCU and CMU at the Manor Hospital, Walsall, for their help with supplying ECGs.

I am grateful to David Richley, Principal Cardiac Physiologist at the James Cook University Hospital in Middlesbrough, for his helpful suggestions to improve the first edition of the book.

Finally, I am grateful to the staff at Wiley-Blackwell for their help, advice and support when preparing the manuscript for the second edition.

*Philip Jevon*

# The Conduction System in the Heart

**1**

## INTRODUCTION

The conduction system in the heart is an intrinsic system whereby the cardiac muscle is automatically stimulated to contract, without the need for external stimulation (Waugh & Grant, 2007). It comprises specialised cardiac cells, which initiate and conduct impulses, providing a stimulus for myocardial contraction. It is controlled by the autonomic nervous system, the sympathetic nerves increase heart rate, contractility, automaticity and atrioventricular (AV) conduction, while the parasympathetic nerves have an opposite effect.

Irregularities in the conduction system can cause cardiac arrhythmias and an abnormal electrocardiogram (ECG). An understanding of the conduction system and how it relates to myocardial contraction and the ECG is essential for ECG interpretation.

The aim of this chapter is to understand the conduction system in the heart.

## LEARNING OUTCOMES

At the end of the chapter the reader will be able to:

❏ Discuss the basic principles of cardiac electrophysiology.
❏ Describe the conduction system in the heart.

## BASIC PRINCIPLES OF CARDIAC ELECTROPHYSIOLOGY

### Depolarisation and repolarisation

The contraction and relaxation of the cardiac muscle results from the depolarisation and repolarisation of myocardial cells (Meek & Morris, 2008):

- *Depolarisation*: can be defined as the sudden surge of charged particles across the membrane of a nerve or muscle cell that accompanies a physicochemical change in the membrane and cancels out or reverses its resting potential to produce an action potential (McFerran & Martin, 2003); put simply, it is the electrical discharging of the cell (Houghton & Gray, 2003). A change in the cell membrane permeability results in electrolyte concentration changes within the cell. This causes the generation of an electrical current, which spreads to neighbouring cells causing these in turn to depolarise. Depolarisation is represented on the ECG as P waves (atrial myocytes) and QRS complexes (ventricular myocytes).

• *Repolarisation*: can be defined as the process by which the cell returns to its normal (resting) electrically charged state after a nerve impulse has passed (McFerran & Martin, 2003); put simply, it is the electrical recharging of the cell (Houghton & Gray, 2003). Ventricular repolarisation is represented on the ECG as T waves (atrial repolarisation is not visible on the ECG as it coincides with and therefore, is masked by the QRS complex).

### Automaticity

Automaticity is the ability of tissue to generate automatically an action potential or current (Marriott & Conover, 1998), i.e. electrical impulses can be generated without any external stimulation. It occurs because there is a small, but constant, leak of positive ions into the cell (Waldo & Wit, 2001).

The sinus node normally has the fastest firing rate and therefore assumes the role of pacemaker for the heart. The speed of automaticity in the SA node can be determined by a number of mechanisms, including the autonomic nervous system and some hormones, e.g. thyroxin (Opie, 1998). If another focus in the heart has a faster firing rate, it will then take over as pacemaker.

### Cardiac action potential

Action potential can be defined as the change in voltage that occurs across the membrane of a muscle or nerve cell when a nerve cell has been triggered (McFarran & Martin, 2003). Cardiac action potential (see Figure 1.1) is the term used to describe the entire sequence of changes in the cell membrane potential, from the beginning of depolarisation to the end of repolarisation.

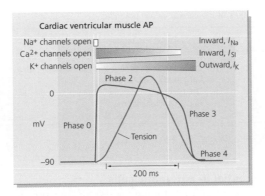

**Figure 1.1** Cardiac ventricular muscle AP. Reprinted from Aaronson, P. & Ward J., *The Cardiovascular System at a Glance*, 3rd edn, copyright 2007, with permission of Blackwell Publishing.

Resting cardiac cells have high potassium and low sodium concentrations (140 mmol/l and 10 mmol/l, respectively). This contrasts sharply with extracellular concentrations (4 mmol/l and 140 mmol/l, respectively) (Jowett & Thompson, 1995). The cell is polarised and has a membrane potential of 90 mV.

Cardiac action potential results from a series of changes in cell permeability to sodium, calcium and potassium ions. Following electrical activation of the cell, a sudden increase in sodium permeability causes a rapid influx of sodium ions into the cell. This is followed by a sustained influx of calcium ions. The membrane potential is now 20 mV. This is referred to as phase 0 of the action potential.

The polarity of the membrane is now slightly positive. As this is the reverse pattern to that of adjacent cells, a potential difference exists, resulting in the flow of electrical current from one cell to the next (Jowett & Thompson, 1995).

The cell returns to its original resting state (repolarisation) (phases 1–3); phase 4 ensues. Sodium is pumped out and potassium and the transmembrane potential returns to its resting of 90 mV. Table 1.1 summarises the phases of the cardiac action potential.

**Table 1.1** Phases of the cardiac action potential.

| Phase | Action |
|-------|--------|
| 0 | Upstroke or spike due to rapid depolarisation |
| 1 | Early rapid depolarisation |
| 2 | The plateau |
| 3 | Rapid repolarisation |
| 4 | Resting membrane potential and diastolic depolarisation |

Thompson 1997

### Action potential in automatic cells

The action potential in automatic cells differs from that in myocardial cells. Automatic cells can initiate an impulse spontaneously without an external impulse.

Automatic cells can be found in the SA node, AV junction (AV node and Bundle of His), bundle branches and Purkinje fibres. The rate of depolarisation varies between the sites:

- *SA node*: has the shortest spontaneous depolarisation time (phase 4) and therefore the quickest firing rate (Julian & Cowan, 1993), usually approximately 60–100 times per minute (Khan, 2004).
- *AV junction (AV node and bundle of His)*: approximately 40–60 times per minute (Sharman, 2007).
- *Bundle branches and Purkinje fibres*: <40 times per minute.

If the SA node firing rate significantly slows or ceases, e.g. a possible complication following an acute inferior myocardial infarction, a subsidiary pacemaker will (it is hoped) provide an escape rhythm. In general, the lower down the conduction system that the pacemaker is sited, the slower the rate, the wider the QRS complex and the less dependable it is (Jowett & Thompson, 1995). When an ectopic pacemaker takes over control of the electrical activity in the heart it is denoted by the prefix 'idio', e.g. an idioventricular rhythm is an escape rhythm originating in the ventricles.

### THE CONDUCTION SYSTEM IN THE HEART

The heart possesses specialised cells that initiate and conduct electrical impulses resulting in myocardial contraction. These

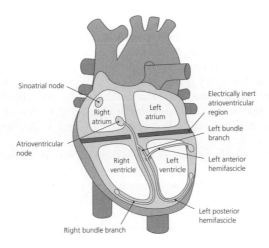

Figure 1.2 The His-Purkinje conduction system. Reprinted from Morris, F. *et al.*, *ABC of Clinical Electrocardiography*, 2nd edn, copyright 2008, with permission of Blackwell Publishing.

cells form the conduction system (see Figure 1.2), which comprises the following:

### Sinoatrial (SA) node

The SA node is situated at the junction of the right atrium and superior vena cava (Sharman, 2007). The blood supply is via the nodal artery, which arises from either the right coronary artery (60%) or the left coronary artery (40%) (Jowett & Thompson, 1995). The SA node acts as the natural pacemaker and initiates each cardiac cycle (Meek & Morris, 2008) and is often referred to as the pacemaker (Khan, 2004; Waugh & Grant, 2007).

### Internodal pathways

The impulse from the SA node is conducted to the atria via four main atrial pathways; three in the right atrium are referred to as internodal pathways because they carry the impulse from the SA node to the AV node (Khan, 2004) and one to the left atrium (Bachmann's bundle) (Berne & Levy, 1992).

## AV node

The AV node is situated near the inferior aspect of the inter-atrial septum (Sharman, 2007). Blood supply is via the nodal artery, which arises from either the right coronary artery (90%) or the left circumflex artery (10%) (Jowett & Thompson, 1995). It acts as a 'bridge' connecting the atria to the ventricles, allowing the impulse to cross the atrioventricular ring (a thick layer of fibrous tissue, which electrically insulates the atria from the ventricles) (Khan, 2004).

The AV node has a slower conduction speed, which delays the conduction of the impulse from the atria to the ventricles (Waldo & Wit, 2001). This allows time for the atria to contract, enabling the ventricles to fill up before contraction (Khan, 2004). Although it does not itself possess the property of automaticity, the AV junction, conduction tissue connecting it to the bundle of His, does (Berne & Levy, 1992).

The AV node has a protective feature, blocking the number of atrial impulses reaching the ventricles (Khan, 2004). This is only seen when the atrial firing rate exceeds 180–200 impulses a minute (Berne & Levy, 1992) which is usually due to an area of abnormal automaticity in the conduction fibres or myocardiam in the atria (Huszar, 2001), e.g. in atrial fibrillation.

## Bundle of His

The bundle of His was first discovered in 1893 by Wilhelm His Jr a Swiss cardiologist and anatomist. It is divided into right and left bundle branches. The left bundle branch is divided into two or sometimes three branches:

- *Anterior fascicle*: radiates anteriorly and superiorly across the ventricular wall.
- *Posterior fascicle*: radiates inferiorly and posteriorly across the left ventricular wall.
- *Mid-septal fascicle*: present in approximately a third of the population (Kulbertus & Demoulin, 1976), it usually emerges directly from the left bundle branch but can arise from either the anterior or posterior fascicle, and radiates through the septum (Dhingra *et al.*, 1975).

(Source: Khan, 2004)

Blood supply is via the left anterior descending artery (Jowett & Thompson, 1995).

### Purkinje fibres

The Purkinje fibres were first discovered in 1839 by the Czech physiologist Johannes Evangelist Purkinje (Purkyne). They form the final part of the conduction system and result from subdivisions of the bundle branches (Sharman, 2007), enabling ventricular contraction from an inward to outward direction (Khan, 2004).

### Control of heart rate

The heart rate is influenced by the cardiovascular centre in the medulla oblongata through the autonomic nervous system (Green, 1991; Waugh & Grant, 2007):

- *Parasympathetic or vagus nerve*: supplies mainly the SA node, AV node and atria (Waugh & Grant, 2007). Continuous vagal activity or vagal tone acts as a brake on the heart. The greater the vagal activity, the slower the heart rate. Increased vagal tone is often associated with an acute inferior myocardial infarction. If vagal activity diminishes, the heart rate will increase. If the vagal tone is completely blocked, the heart rate would be approximately 150 beats per minute (Green, 1991). Atropine blocks the action of the vagus nerve. This causes an increase in heart rate.
- *Sympathetic nerve*: supplies the SA node, AV node, atria and ventricles (Waugh & Grant, 2007). Sympathetic nerve activity ('fight and flight') has a positive chronotropic action on the heart, i.e. it increases the heart rate. It is particularly active in periods of emotional excitement, exercise and stress. Beta blockers shield the heart from sympathetic nerve activity resulting in a decrease in heart rate, blood pressure and myocardial workload.

## CHAPTER SUMMARY

The conduction system in the heart comprises specialised cardiac cells, which initiate and conduct impulses, providing a stimulus for myocardial contraction. This chapter has provided an overview to the conduction system. The basic principles of cardiac electrophysiology have been discussed. The conduction system has been described together with how the ECG relates to cardiac contraction.

## REFERENCES

Berne R, Levy M (1992) *Cardiovascular Physiology*, 6th edn. Mosby, St Louis.

Dhingra R, Wyndam C, Ehsani A, Rosen K (1975) Electrocardiogram of the month: left anterior hemiblock concealing diaphragmatic infarction and simulating anteroseptal infarction. *Chest*, **67**, 713–715.

Green J (1991) *An Introduction to Human Physiology*. Oxford Medical Publications, Oxford.

Houghton A, Gray D (2003) *Making Sense of the ECG: a Hands on Guide*, 2nd edn. Hodder Arnold, London.

Huszar J (2001) *Basic Dysrhythmias: Interpretation and Management*, 3rd edn. Mosby, St Louis.

Jowett NI, Thompson DR (1995) *Comprehensive Coronary Care*, 2nd edn. Scutari Press, London.

Julian D, Cowan J (1993) *Cardiology*, 6th edn. Baillière, London.

Khan E (2004) Clinical skills: the physiological basis and interpretation of the ECG. *British Journal of Nursing*, **13** (8), 440–446.

Kulbertus H, Demoulin J (1976) Pathological basis of concept left hemiblock. In: Wellens H, Lie K, Janse M (eds) *The Conduction System of the Heart*. Lea and Febiger, Philadelphia.

McFerran T, Martin E (2003) *Minidictionary for Nurses*, 5th edn, Oxford University Press, Oxford.

Marriott H, Conover M (1998) *Advanced Concepts in Arrhythmias*, 3rd edn. Mosby, St Louis.

Meek S, Morris F (2008) Introduction. 1-leads, rate, rhythm and cardiac axis. In: Morris F, Brady W, Camm J (eds) *ABC of Clinical Electrocardiography*, 2nd edn. Blackwell Publishing, Oxford.

Opie L (1998) *The Heart: Physiology from Cell lo Circulation*, 3rd edn. Lippincott Williams & Wilkins, Philadelphia.

Sharman J (2007) Clinical skills: cardiac rhythm recognition and monitoring. *British Journal of Nursing*, **16** (5), 307.

Thompson P (1997) *Coronary Care Manual*. Churchill Livingstone, London.

Hurst J (1998) Naming of the waves in the ECG, with a brief account of their genesis. *Circulation*, **98**, 1937–1942.

Sykes A, Waller A (1887) The electrocardiogram. *BMJ (Clin Res Ed)*, **294**, 1396–1398.

Snellen H (1995) *Willem Einthoven (1860–1927): Father of Electrocardiography*. Kluwer Academic Publishers, Dordrecht, Netherlands.

Waldo L, Wit A (2001) Mechanisms of cardiac arrhythmias and conduction disturbance. In: Fuster V, Alexander R, O'Rourke R, *et al.* (eds) *Hurst's the Heart*. McGraw Hill, New York.

Waller A (1887) A demonstration on man of electromotive changes accompanying the heart's beat. *J Physiol*, **8**, 229–234.

Waugh A, Grant A (2007) *Ross and Wilson Anatomy and Physiology in Health and Illness*, 10th edn (reprint). Elsevier, Edinburgh.

# 2 | Principles of ECG Monitoring

## INTRODUCTION

An electrocardiogram (ECG) (*electro* – relating to or caused by electricity, *cardio* – from the Greek word kardia 'heart' and gram – from the Greek word gramma 'thing written') can be defined as a record or display of a person's heartbeat produced by electrocardiography (Soanes & Stevenson, 2006).

Electrocardiography is the measurement of electrical activity in the heart (using an electrocardiograph, e.g. cardiac monitor, ECG machine) and recording it as a visual trace, either on paper or on an oscilloscope screen, by placing electrodes on the skin (Soanes & Stevenson, 2006).

ECG monitoring is one of the most valuable diagnostic tools in modern medicine (Drew *et al.*, 2005). The goals of ECG monitoring in hospital settings have expanded from simple heart rate and basic rhythm interpretation to the diagnosis of complex cardiac arrhythmias, myocardial ischaemia and prolonged QT interval (Drew *et al.*, 2005).

ECG monitoring must be meticulously undertaken. Potential consequences of poor technique include misinterpretation of cardiac arrhythmias, mistaken diagnosis, wasted investigations and mismanagement of the patient (Drew *et al.*, 2005).

The aim of this chapter is to understand the principles of ECG monitoring.

## LEARNING OUTCOMES

At the end of the chapter the reader will be able to:

❑ Outline the historical background to ECG monitoring.
❑ Discuss how the ECG relates to cardiac contraction.

❏ List the indications for ECG monitoring.
❏ State the common features of a cardiac monitor.
❏ Describe the positioning of ECG electrodes.
❏ Describe the procedure for cardiac monitoring.
❏ Discuss the problems associated with cardiac monitoring.
❏ Outline the principles of exercise testing.

## HISTORICAL BACKGROUND TO ECG MONITORING
### Invention of the ECG

The current generated by the conduction system in the heart was first recorded in humans by Augustus Waller at St Mary's Hospital, London, in 1887 (Waller, 1887). He had used a Lippmann capillary electrometer, which had revealed two deflections: he labelled these two waves V1 and V2 according to the anatomical parts of the heart that had produced them (i.e. ventricles) (Hurst, 1998). Unfortunately, Waller did not recognise the clinical importance and significance of his discovery (Sykes & Waller, 1887).

It fell to Willem Einthoven from The Netherlands to refine Waller's techniques in the early 1900's and generate a clinically relevant ECG (Hurst, 1998; Khan, 2004). It is for this reason that Einthoven is generally recognised as the father of ECG (Khan, 2004; Snellen, 1995).

Using a Lippmann capillary electrometer, Einthoven also recorded two waves generated by the ventricles, but originally labelled them A and B; when he subsequently recorded a wave generated by the atria, he labelled it P after Descartes' use of the letter P to designate a point on a curve (René Descartes was a seventeenth century French philosopher and mathematician, who invented analytical geometry and used the letters PQRST to denote points on curves he drew) (Hurst, 1998).

Einthoven subsequently used PQRST to label the waves, which is still in use today (Snellen, 1995). It has been suggested that Einthoven chose the letters from the centre of the alphabet because he did not know whether other waves preceding the P wave and following the T wave would be subsequently discovered as recording instruments improved (Hurst, 1998); in fact, he subsequently discovered the U wave a few years later (Snellen, 1995).

**Brief history of coronary care units**

The emergence of cardiopulmonary resuscitation (CPR) and defibrillation in the 1960s led to the introduction of hospital coronary care units in Kansas City (Day, 1963) and Toronto (Brown *et al.*, 1963). The aim of these first coronary care units (CCUs) was to reduce mortality from acute myocardial infarction (AMI) (Quinn & Thompson, 1999). Pioneering cardiologists recognised the threat of cardiac arrest due to malignant arrhythmias in the post-myocardial infarction setting, and developed techniques for successful external defibrillation (Khush *et al.*, 2005).

The experience of hospital coronary care units demonstrated that the majority of deaths occurred from ventricular fibrillation, a treatable arrhythmia (Pantridge & Wilson, 1996). Arrhythmia monitoring, CPR and defibrillation were performed by coronary care trained nursing staff, thus eliminating delays in treatment and significantly reducing mortality. It was claimed that coronary care units reduced the hospital mortality from 30% to 20% (Pantridge, 1970).

However, most of the deaths complicating acute myocardial infarction occurred in the community. Researchers in Seattle reported that 63% of deaths from coronary heart disease in persons <50 years of age occurred within one hour of the onset of symptoms (Bainton & Peterson, 1963).This was recognised by Pantridge, a pioneering Belfast cardiologist, who in 1965 established a mobile coronary care ambulance equipped with the world's first portable defibrillator.

These early triumphs in aborting sudden death led to the development of techniques to treat cardiogenic shock, limit myocardial infarct size and initiate pre-hospital coronary care, all of which laid the foundation for the current era of interventional cardiology (Khush *et al.*, 2005). ECG monitoring is still a fundamental part of coronary care nursing today, just as it was in the 1960s.

## HOW THE ECG RELATES TO CARDIAC CONTRACTION

Figure 2.1 depicts how the ECG relates to cardiac contraction and is as follows:

(1) The SA node fires and the electrical impulse spreads across the atria, resulting in atrial contraction (P wave).

(2) On arriving at the AV node the impulse is delayed, allowing the atria time to fully contract and eject blood into the ventricles. This brief period of absent electrical activity is represented on the ECG by a straight (isoelectric) line between the end of the P wave and the beginning of the QRS complex. The PR interval represents atrial depolarisation and the impulse delay in the AV node prior to ventricular depolarisation.

(3) The impulse is then conducted down to the ventricles through the bundle of His, right and left bundle branches and Purkinje fibres causing ventricular depolarisation and contraction (QRS complex).

(4) The ventricles then repolarise (T wave).

**Sinus rhythm**

Sinus rhythm (shown in Figure 2.2) is the normal rhythm of the heart. The impulse originates in the SA node (i.e. 'sinus') at a regular rate of 60–100 per minute. Each impulse is conducted down the normal pathways to the ventricles without any abnormal conduction delays. It may sometimes present as a cardiac arrest, but without a resultant cardiac output (pulseless electrical activity) (see page 164).

Identifying features on the ECG:

- *Electrical activity*: present.
- *QRS rate*: 60–100 per min.
- *QRS rhythm*: regular.
- *QRS width*: normal width and morphology.
- *P waves*: present and of constant morphology.
- *Relationship between P waves and QRS complexes*: each P wave is followed by a QRS complex and each QRS complex is proceeded by a P wave. PR interval normal and constant.

## INDICATIONS FOR ECG MONITORING

Since the introduction of ECG monitoring in hospital and the establishment of coronary care units in the 1960s (Day, 1963), the goals of monitoring have expanded from simple heart rate and basic rhythm monitoring to the diagnosis of complex arrhythmias, the detection of myocardial ischaemia, and the identification of a prolonged QT interval (Drew *et al.*, 2005).

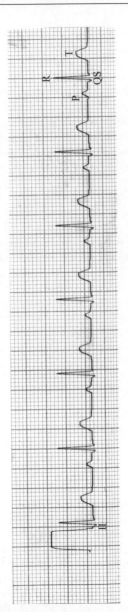

**Figure 2.1** The ECG and its relation to cardiac contraction.

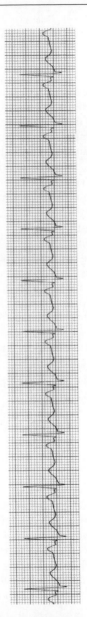

**Figure 2.2** Sinus rhythm.

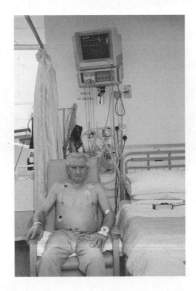

**Figure 2.3** ECG monitoring.

ECG monitoring (see Figure 2.3) has seen major developments, including computerised arrhythmia detection algorithms, ST-segment/ischaemia monitoring software, improved noise reduction strategies, multilead monitoring, and reduced lead sets for monitoring derived 12 lead ECGs with a minimal number of electrodes (Dower *et al.*, 1988; Drew *et al.*, 2002; 2005).

Myocardial ischaemia is now aggressively treated; strategies to prevent infarction or to reduce infarct size rely heavily on healthcare professionals being able to identify myocardial ischaemia in emergency departments and to provide ongoing close monitoring to detect recurrent ischaemia in coronary care units etc. (Drew *et al.*, 2005).

The introduction of electrophysiological interventions, e.g. catheter ablation, biventricular pacing and implantable cardioverter defibrillators, requires healthcare professionals to be able to analyse ECG monitoring data for evidence of device malfunction and suboptimal device programming (Drew *et al.*, 2005).

Drugs have been introduced that can cause prolongation of ventricular repolarisation; healthcare professionals need to be able to recognise a prolonged QT interval. Failure to do so could result in malignant ventricular arrhythmias, e.g. torsades de pointes (Drew *et al.*, 2005).

## American College of Cardiology guidelines

The American College of Cardiology Emergency Cardiac Care Committee has devised the following classification for indications for ECG monitoring:

- Class I: ECG monitoring is indicated in most, if not all, patients in this group.
- Class II: ECG monitoring may be of benefit in some patients but is not considered essential for all patients.
- Class III: ECG monitoring is not indicated because a patient's risk of a serious event is so low that monitoring has no therapeutic benefit.

(Mirvis *et al.*, 1989)

## Class I group of patients

These patients are at significant risk of developing a life-threatening cardiac arrhythmia and include:

- Post-successful cardiopulmonary resuscitation.
- Acute coronary syndromes.
- Newly diagnosed high-risk coronary lesions.
- Following cardiac surgery.
- Following cardiac pacing.
- Second or third degree AV block.
- Long-QT syndrome and associated ventricular arrhythmias.
- During intra-aortic balloon counterpulsation.
- Acute heart failure.
- Transfer to intensive care.
- During diagnostic/therapeutic procedures requiring conscious sedation or anaesthesia.
- Drug overdose (if there is a risk of pro-arrhythmic complications).

(Sources: Drew *et al.*, 2005; Jevon, 2006)

## Class II group of patients

ECG monitoring may be beneficial in some, but not all, of the following patients:

- Post-acute myocardial infarction: whether to continue monitoring acute MI patients from 24 to 48 hours following admission is controversial (Drew *et al.*, 2005).
- Chest pain, but no diagnostic EGG findings or elevated biomarkers.
- Receiving anti-arrhythmic drug therapy for chronic atrial fibrillation when it is being titrated according to the response.
- Following the insertion of a permanent pacemaker, but is not pacemaker dependent.
- Following uncomplicated catheter ablation.
- Post-routine coronary angiography.
- Heart failure.
- History of syncope.
- Do Not Attempt Resuscitate order in place, but patient has a cardiac arrhythmia causing him discomfort.

(Sources: Drew *et al.*, 2005; Jevon, 2006)

## Class III group of patients

ECG monitoring is not indicated in this group of patients because the risk of a serious event is so low that monitoring has no therapeutic benefit. There are many such situations including:

- Post-uncomplicated surgical procedures in patients who are at low risk for cardiac arrhythmias.
- Obstetric patients, unless there is existing heart disease.
- Permanent, rate-controlled atrial fibrillation.

(Sources: Drew *et al.*, 2005; Jevon, 2006)

## COMMON FEATURES OF A CARDIAC MONITOR

The bedside cardiac monitor (see Figure 2.4) or oscilloscope provides a continuous display of the patient's ECG and has the following common features:

- *Screen for displaying the ECG trace*, a dull/bright switch can be adjusted if the screen is too light or too dark.

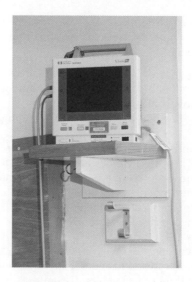

**Figure 2.4** Bedside cardiac monitor.

- *ECG printout facility*, to record cardiac arrhythmias (invaluable for both diagnosis and record keeping purposes).
- *Heart rate counter*, to calculate the heart rate (counts the QRS complexes).
- *Monitor alarms*, to alert the healthcare professional to changes in heart rate to outside pre-set limits. Some cardiac monitors can identify important cardiac arrhythmias and changes in the ST segment, and alarm accordingly.
- *Lead select switch*, to select the desired monitoring lead, e.g. lead II.
- *ECG gain*, to alter the size of the ECG complex. If it is set too low or too high the ECG trace can become unrecognisable, either too small or distorted, leading to the possibility of misinterpretation (see Figure 2.5).

## POSITIONING OF ECG ELECTRODES
An electrode can be defined as a conductor through which electrical current enters or leaves an object (Soanes & Stevenson, 2006).

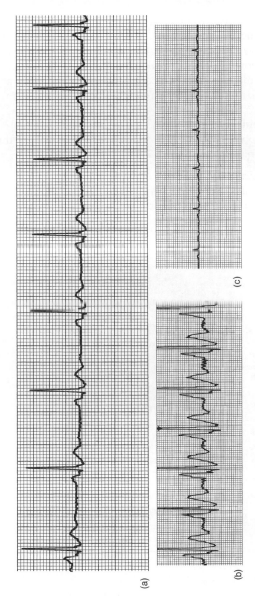

(a)

(b)

(c)

**Figure 2.5** Effects of incorrect ECG gain setting. (a) 10 mm/1 mV – standard setting; ECG complexes adequate size. (b) 40 mm/1 mV – ECG complexes too large; cardiac monitor mistook the P and T waves for QRS complexes, resulting in continuous false-high heart rate alarms. (c) 2 mm/1 mV – ECG complexes too small; cardiac monitor did not recognise QRS complexes, resulting in continuous false asystole alarms. Also difficulties may be encountered interpreting cardiac arrhythmias when the gain is set too low.

The correct positioning of ECG electrodes is crucial for obtaining accurate information from any monitoring lead (Jacobson, 2000). Whether a three or a five ECG cable monitoring system is used will depend upon the patient, the desired monitoring lead(s), local protocols, the manufacturer's recommendations and what actually needs to be monitored, e.g. cardiac arrhythmias, ST segment.

### Three ECG cable system

The standard positioning of ECG electrodes when using a three ECG cable monitoring system is:

- *Red ECG cable*: below the right clavicle.
- *Yellow ECG cable*: below the left clavicle.
- *Green ECG cable*: left lower thorax/hip region.

This is shown in Figure 2.6.

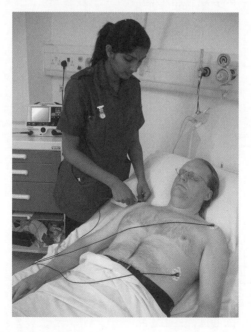

**Figure 2.6** Three ECG cable system.

These bipolar leads, which record the potential difference between two electrodes, can be used to monitor lead I, lead II, lead III or a modified chest lead such as MCL1 (Drew *et al.*, 2005).

Bipolar lead monitoring can be used to track heart rate, for basic arrhythmia monitoring, to detect R waves for synchronised electrical cardioversion and to detect ventricular fibrillation (Drew *et al.*, 2005). Lead II is usually selected (Resuscitation Council UK, 2006).

However, this type of monitoring is inadequate for sophisticated monitoring of cardiac arrhythmias because it doesn't contain lead V1 (Drew *et al.*, 2005). Lead V1 is considered the best lead for diagnosing right and left bundle-branch block, to confirm proper right ventricular pacemaker location in temporary transvenous pacing, and to distinguish between ventricular tachycardia and supraventricular tachycardia with aberrant conduction (Drew *et al.*, 2005).

Some clinical areas prefer to monitor on MCL1 (modified chest lead 1, i.e. bipolar substitute for V1) as recommended by Marriott (1988). The positioning of ECG electrodes is:

- *Black ECG cable*: right shoulder.
- *Red ECG cable*: left shoulder.
- *Yellow ECG cable*: fourth intercostal space, just to the right of the sternum, i.e. corresponding to V1.

However, the reliability of QRS morphology using MCL1 monitoring has been questioned (60% accuracy); it is therefore not recommended for diagnosing wide QRS complex tachycardia (Drew & Scheinman, 1995).

**Five ECG cable system**
ECG monitoring using a five ECG cable system is becoming more popular. The main advantage of this system is that different ECG leads can be monitored simultaneously. This is particularly useful when analysing cardiac arrhythmias and ST segments as it provides an alternative view of the waveform. Cardiac monitors with this lead system often have two channels for ECG display, i.e. one limb lead and one precordial lead can be displayed simultaneously (Drew *et al.*, 2005).

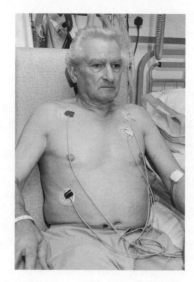

**Figure 2.7** Five ECG cable system.

The standard positioning for ECG electrodes is illustrated in Figure. 2.7 and is as follows:

- *RA (red ECG cable)*: below the right clavicle.
- *LA (yellow ECG cable)*: below the left clavicle.
- *RL (black ECG cable)*: right lower thorax/hip region.
- *LL (green ECG cable)*: left lower thorax/hip region.
- *(white ECG cable)*: on the chest in the desired V position, usually V1 (4th intercostal space just right of the sternum. NB in Figure 2.7 the V2 position has been utilised).

(Drew *et al.*, 2005)

### Ten cable Mason-Likar 12 lead ECG system

In 1966, Mason and Likar proposed a variation on the positioning of the standard limb electrodes (chest electrodes to remain in the standard position), when undertaking 12 lead ECG exercise stress testing (Mason & Likar, 1966). Instead of attaching wires to the wrists and ankles, where excessive movement during exercise testing could result in interference and unreadable ECG traces (limb leads), they suggested:

- *RA (red ECG cable)*: right infraclavicular fossa medial to the border of the deltoid muscle.
- *LA (yellow ECG cable)*: left infraclavicular fossa medial to the border of the deltoid muscle.
- *RL (black ECG cable)*: left iliac fossa.
- *LL (green ECG cable)*: anywhere, but usually right iliac fossa.

(Source: Drew *et al.*, 2005)

The above configuration is frequently used when undertaking ECG monitoring using a five cable system (see above). The disadvantage of the Mason-Likar lead system for ECG monitoring is that ten electrodes are required and the six precordial electrodes often interfere with diagnostic (e.g. echocardiograms, chest X-rays) and emergency (defibrillation sites) procedures. In addition, the precordial sites are difficult to maintain in women with large breasts and men with hairy chests (Drew *et al.*, 2005).

### EASI 12 lead ECG monitoring

The conventional 12 lead ECG using ten electrodes attached to the limbs and chest is recognised as the current medical standard for the identification, analysis and confirmation of many cardiac abnormalities, including cardiac arrhythmias and cardiac ischaemia/infarction. If 12 lead ECG monitoring is undertaken on a continual basis, the benefits include:

- Facilitating the accurate recognition of cardiac arrhythmias.
- Enabling the monitoring of the mid-precordial leads, which is particularly important for the detection and management of ischaemia.
- Enabling the recording of *transient* ECG events of particular diagnostic or therapeutic importance.
- Enabling the differentiation between post-PTCA ischaemia and occlusion.

Unfortunately, the use of a conventional 12 lead ECG system using ten electrodes for continuous cardiac monitoring is cumbersome and generally not practical in the clinical area. However, the EASI system, a new concept in 12 lead ECG monitoring, requires the use of only five electrodes:

- *E* electrode on the lower sternum at the level of the fifth intercostal space.
- *A* on the left midaxillary line on the same level as the E electrode.
- *S* electrode on the upper sternum.
- *I* on the right midaxillary line on the same level as the E electrode.

A fifth ground electrode can be placed anywhere. The system is illustrated in Figure 2.8.

The EASI system for 12 lead ECG (Philips) monitoring using only five electrodes is less cumbersome and more practical than

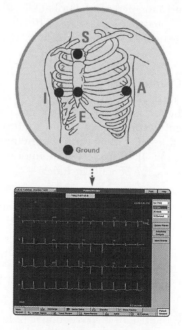

**Figure 2.8** EASI system for 12 lead ECG monitoring system. Reproduced by kind permission of Philips Healthcare.

the standard ten electrode system. It is therefore more comfortable for the patient. In addition it will not interfere with such procedures as cardiac auscultation, CPR, defibrillation and echocardiography.

### Selection of ECG monitoring leads

When undertaking cardiac monitoring to diagnose cardiac arrhythmias or to detect changes in the cardiac axis, it is important to select an ECG monitoring lead that clearly displays atrial and ventricular activity. The R wave configuration should be at least double the amplitude of the T wave, so that the heart rate will be accurately displayed and computer rhythm analysis will be correct (Thompson, 1997).

Lead II provides upright positive waveforms with good visualisation of the P waves. It is used for analysing atrial arrhythmias, differentiating between atrial and junctional arrhythmias, AV blocks and atrial pacing. It is recommended during cardiopulmonary resuscitation. Lead II can be viewed using either of the above ECG electrode positions.

MCL1 (modified chest lead, V1) enables differentiation between ventricular and supraventricular arrhythmias and identification of bundle branch blocks (Meltzer *et al.*, 1983). However, it does not enable the recognition of changes in the cardiac axis. MCL1 can be viewed using the ECG electrode position described for the five ECG cable monitoring system or with a modified ECG electrode position for using a three ECG cable system.

## PROCEDURE TO ESTABLISH ECG MONITORING

ECG monitoring is performed in a wide variety of clinical settings, including critical care, coronary care, A & E, acute medical/ surgical wards, high risk obstetric cases, cardiac catheterisation, theatre and recovery. The goals and methods of ECG monitoring can differ, e.g. in A & E, ST segment monitoring is important in acute coronary care syndromes (Drew *et al.*, 2005), i.e. an appropriate monitoring system will be required, such as five cable or EASI system (see above).

Correct electrode placement and adequate skin preparation are important to ensure an accurate and reliable ECG trace (Sharman, 2007). Examples of incorrect treatment due to inaccurate or poor

ECG monitoring techniques have been reported in the literature, e.g. unnecessary cardiac catheterisation because of false ST-segment monitor alarms (Drew *et al.*, 2001), unnecessary electrophysiology testing and device implantation because of muscle artefact simulating ventricular tachycardia (Knight *et al.*, 1999).

A suggested procedure to establish ECG monitoring is as follows:

(1) Ascertain why ECG monitoring is required.
(2) Explain the procedure to the patient, as it can be quite daunting (Sharman, 2007).
(3) If necessary, carefully shave the chest to remove excess chest hair (Drew *et al.*, 2005) (always obtain patient consent first), as this will help ensure better contact and also make it less uncomfortable for the patient when removing the ECG electrodes (Perez, 1996). Care should be taken when shaving, because if the skin is grazed there is a risk of infection (because of this some authorities suggest cutting chest hair instead of shaving) (Sharman, 2007).
(4) Reduce skin oil and debris by gently rubbing the skin with alcohol or some gauze (see Figure 2.9) (Navas, 2003). Mild abrasion of the skin will reduce impedance between the skin and electrode, thus reducing interference (Thompson, 1997). Some clinical areas use a specially designed material to do this.

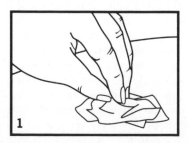

**Figure 2.9** Establishing ECG monitoring: prepare the chest. Reproduced by kind permission of Ambu.

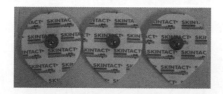

**Figure 2.10** ECG electrode. Reproduced by kind permission of Ambu.

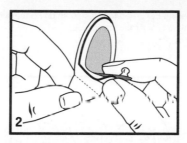

**Figure 2.11** Establishing ECG monitoring: remove the backing from the ECG electrodes. Reproduced by kind permission of Ambu.

(5) Ensure the skin is dry. This will help the ECG electrodes to adhere to the skin.

(6) Check the ECG electrodes (see Figure 2.10). They should be in date and still moist, not dry.

(7) Remove the protective backing from the ECG electrodes and expose the gel disc (see Figure 2.11).

(8) Apply the ECG electrodes to the patient's chest following locally agreed protocols. The electrodes should lie flat. If the electrodes have an offset connector (to absorb tugs) these should be pointed towards the ECG cables.

(9) Smooth down the adhesive area with a circular motion (see Figure 2.12). Avoid pressing on the gel disc itself as this may result in a decrease in electrode conductivity and adherence (Thompson, 1997).

(10) Attach the ECG cables to the electrodes (see Figure 2.13). (NB If 'snap-on' ECG cables are being used with central

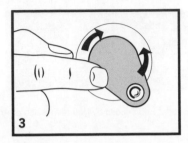

**Figure 2.12** Establishing ECG monitoring: smooth down the adhesive area. Reproduced by kind permission of Ambu.

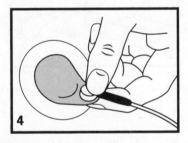

**Figure 2.13** Establishing ECG monitoring: attach the ECG cables to the electrodes. Reproduced by kind permission of Ambu.

stud electrodes, connect them up before application to the patient's skin.).

(11) Switch the cardiac monitor on and select the required monitoring ECG lead.

(12) Ensure the ECG trace is clear. Rectify any difficulties encountered (see below).

(13) Set the alarms within safe parameters following locally agreed protocols and appropriate to the patient's clinical condition (Docherty, 2003; Drew *et al.*, 2005). The alarm settings are usually set at <50/min and >120/min (Docherty, 2003).

(14) Anchor the ECG cables. They should not be allowed to pull on the ECG electrodes.
(15) Position the cardiac monitor so it is clearly visible.
(16) Document in the patient's notes that cardiac monitoring has commenced and the ECG rhythm identified.
(17) Regularly monitor the electrode sites for signs of allergy – redness, itching and erythema. ECG electrodes should be regularly replaced (Sharman, 2007). (Main source for this text: Jevon, 2006).

### Infection control issues

There is a potential risk for infection from reusable ECG wires that are poorly decontaminated between patients (Brown, 2006). Contaminated ECG wires had previously been cited as a source of an outbreak of vancomycin-resistant enterococci (Falk *et al.*, 2000). In a small study, 77% of supposedly clean wires were found to be contaminated with antibiotic-resistant bacteria (Jancin, 2004).

It is important to ensure that local infection control policies advise on how to clean wires after use; for example, using a hospital-grade disinfectant according to manufacturer's instructions (Houghton, 2006).

### Telemetry

Telemetry (see Figure 2.14) is a convenient method of monitoring the ECG while the patient is mobilising. ECG electrodes are connected to a small portable transmitter, which the patient carries around in a pyjama pocket or pouch.

The radio signals are transmitted to a central console (normally on CCU) (see Figure 2.15) where any important cardiac arrhythmias can be identified. The advantage of this system is that patients can be mobilised in the early period following a myocardial infarction yet still benefit from close cardiac monitoring (Jowett & Thompson, 1995). It also frees up monitored CCU beds (Thompson, 1997).

### Ambulatory cardiac monitoring (24-hour tape)

There are limitations to ECG monitoring when investigating paroxysmal cardiac arrhythmias (Kennedy, 1992). To overcome

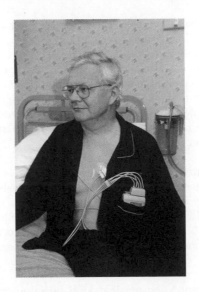

**Figure 2.14** Telemetry.

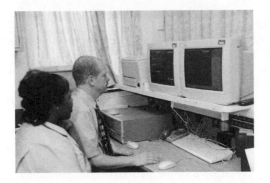

**Figure 2.15** Central console.

these, ambulatory cardiac monitoring has been developed (Petch, 1985).

Ambulatory cardiac monitoring is designed to identify transient disturbances in the ECG rhythm, rate and conduction, together with any associated symptoms (DiMarco & Philbrick, 1990). It can help to assess the effectiveness of anti-arrhythmic drug therapy, detect ischaemia and determine prognosis (Mickley, 1994).

The patient is asked to continue with normal daily activities. A patient diary should be kept and any episodes of pain, dizziness, palpitations, syncope, etc., together with exact timings, should be recorded. Some machines have an 'event marker' button which the patient can press at the onset of symptoms.

A typical 24-hour tape will record 100,000 QRS complexes for analysis. Fortunately, high-speed electrocardioscanners are able to replay the tape in a matter of minutes (Jowett & Thompson, 1995). Areas of interest can be printed out, particularly ECG strips during periods when the patient experienced symptoms.

Best practice ECG monitoring includes the following:

- Ensure adequate skin preparation.
- Use ECG electrodes that are in date with moist gel sponge.
- Position ECG electrodes and select monitoring lead following locally agreed protocols.
- Set cardiac monitor alarms according to the patient's clinical condition.
- Ensure the ECG trace is accurate.
- Ensure the cardiac monitor is visible.

## PROBLEMS ASSOCIATED WITH ECG MONITORING

There are numerous problems associated with ECG monitoring; some are due to the limitations of the monitoring system itself, whereas others are due to poor technique (Meltzer *et al.*, 1983). Potential problems that may be encountered are described below.

### 'Flat line' trace

Check the patient! The most likely cause is mechanical. Check that the:

- Correct ECG monitoring lead is selected (usually lead II).
- ECG gain is set correctly.
- Electrodes are in date and the gel sponge is moist, not dry.
- ECG cables are properly connected to the electrodes.
- ECG cables are not broken and are plugged into the monitor.

**Poor quality ECG trace**
If the ECG trace quality is poor, check the:

- Connections.
- Brightness display.
- Electrodes are in date and that the gel sponge is moist, not dry (Perez, 1996).
- Electrodes are properly attached.

If there are still difficulties obtaining a clear ECG trace, wiping the skin with an alcohol swab may help. If the patient is sweating profusely, the application of a small amount of tincture benzoin to the skin, leaving it to dry before applying the electrodes, is recommended (Jowett & Thompson, 1995). As electrodes tend to dry out after about three days, they should be changed at least that often, though every 24 hours may be optimum to maintain skin integrity (Perez, 1996).

**Voluntary patient movement artefact or wandering ECG baseline**
Voluntary patient movement artefact or wandering ECG baseline (ECG trace going up and down) (see Figure 2.16) is usually

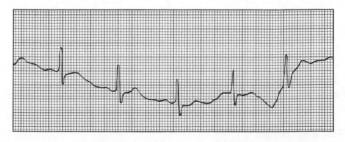

**Figure 2.16** Voluntary patient movement artefact. Reproduced by kind permission of Ambu.

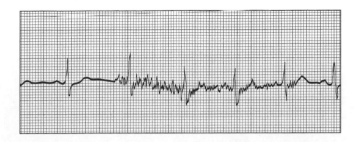

**Figure 2.17** Involuntary patient movement artefact. Reproduced by kind permission of Ambu.

caused by patient movement, particularly by respiration. If respiration is the cause and the problem is not transient, reposition the electrodes away from the lower ribs (Meltzer *et al.*, 1983). If it occurs in obese patients, it is difficult to correct.

### Involuntary patient movement artefact
Involuntary patient movement artefact is usually caused by a tremor, e.g. if the patient is cold or nervous (see Figure 2.17). The patient should be reassured and kept warm. If the patient has a tremor associated with Parkinson's disease, very little can be done to remedy the artefact.

### Electrical interference
Electrical interference, e.g. from bedside infusion pumps, can cause a 'fuzzy' appearance on the ECG trace, making it difficult to interpret. Remove the source of the interference if possible.

### Loose electrode
A wandering baseline, together with sudden breaks in the signal (see Figure 2.10), often indicates a loose electrode. Causes include incorrect positioning, e.g. over a joint, and poor electrode site, e.g. hairy skin or dry, not moist electrode.

### Small ECG complexes
Sometimes the ECG complexes may be too small and unrecognisable (see Figure 2.5). Possible causes include pericardial effusion,

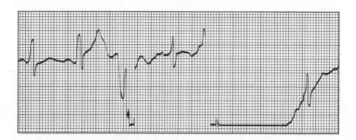

**Figure 2.18** Loose electrode. Reproduced by kind permission of Ambu.

obesity and hypothyroidism. However, sometimes a technical problem is the cause. Check that the ECG gain is correctly set and the desired ECG monitoring lead has been selected; repositioning the electrodes or selecting another ECG monitoring lead sometimes helps.

### Incorrect heart rate display
If the ECG complexes are too small, a false-low heart rate may be displayed. Large T waves (see Figure 2.5), muscle movement and interference can be mistaken for QRS complexes, resulting in a false-high heart rate being displayed. The nurse must be alert to the possibility of inaccurate heart rate readings, especially those that might be caused by poor electrode contact and interference (Ren *et al.*, 1998). To minimise the potential for inaccuracies, a good quality ECG trace should be obtained.

### False alarms
Frequent false alarms will undermine the rationale for setting alarms and will cause undue anxiety for the patient. It is important to ensure that the alarms are correctly and appropriately set. An accurate ECG trace will reduce the frequency of false alarms. A poor connection (see Figure 2.19) can also lead to false alarms.

### Skin irritation
ECG electrodes can cause skin irritation. The electrode sites should be regularly examined for redness, itching and erythema.

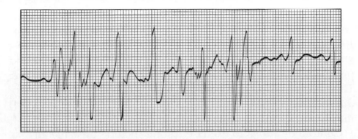

**Figure 2.19** Poor electrode contact. Reproduced by kind permission of Ambu.

If the patient's skin appears irritated, select another site for electrode placement (Paul & Hebra, 1998). If necessary, use hypoallergenic ECG electrodes (Thompson, 1997). Regularly replace the ECG electrodes (Sharman, 2007).

### PRINCIPLES OF EXERCISE STRESS TESTING
Exercise stress testing, first introduced in the 1940s (Master *et al.*, 1942), has traditionally been used for the diagnosis of coronary artery disease. However, it is now equally important in the assessment of patients with known disease (Detry & Fox, 1996).

It provides an accurate physiological evaluation of coronary flow reserve, which, in terms of prognosis, becomes more significant than simply the number of anatomical lesions (Detry & Fox, 1996).

The main aims of exercise testing are to:

• Provoke symptoms, e.g. chest pain and dyspnoea.
• Identify ECG changes associated with progressive workload.
• Determine maximum workload.
• Assess prognosis.

(Jowett & Thompson, 1995)

Generally the early onset of angina with significant and widespread ST depression, slow recovery and a poor blood pressure response are indicative of severe coronary artery disease (Jowett & Thompson, 1995).

There are numerous exercise protocols available for diagnostic and prognostic assessment during exercise testing (Detry & Fox, 1996). However, the Bruce protocol (Bruce *et al.*, 1963) is the most widely used (Detry & Fox, 1996). It is suitable for routine use and produces a rapid increase in progressive workload (Jowett & Thompson, 1995). For patients with known coronary artery disease, the slower Naughton protocol (Naughton *et al.*, 1964) may be better suited (Jowett & Thompson, 1995).

Contraindications to exercise testing include unstable angina, severe hypertension, anaemia, electrolyte imbalances and serious cardiac arrhythmias (Jowett & Thompson, 1995). As life-threatening cardiac arrhythmias, e.g. ventricular fibrillation, can occur during the test (Irving *et al.*, 1977), it is important to ensure that adequate resuscitation facilities are available. National guidelines are available when undertaking exercise testing without direct medical supervision (British Cardiac Society, 1993).

**Myoview stress test**

Myoview stress tests using adenosine or dobutamine are ideal for patients who are unable to tolerate going on a treadmill. The drug is administered intravenously to simulate a stress condition on the heart by vasodilation. Resultant myocardial ischaemia is assessed by differences in uptake of a radio-isotope in addition to 12 lead ECG monitoring.

CHAPTER SUMMARY

This chapter has provided an overview to the principles of ECG monitoring. The indications for cardiac monitoring, common features of a cardiac monitor, ECG electrode placement, procedure for cardiac monitoring together with problems associated and what the ECG trace records, have been discussed.

ECG monitoring must be meticulously undertaken. Consequences of poor technique could include misinterpretation of cardiac arrhythmias, mistaken diagnosis, wasted investigations and mismanagement of the patient.

REFERENCES

Bainton C, Peterson D (1963) Deaths from coronary heart disease in persons 50 years of age and younger. *N Engl J Med*, **268**, 569–575.

British Cardiac Society (1993) Guidelines on exercise testing when there is not a doctor present. *British Heart Journal*, **70**, 488.

Brown D (2006) Electrocardiography wires: a potential source of infection *AACN News*, **23** (9),12–15.

Brown K, MacMillan R, Forbath N, *et al.* (1963) Coronary unit: an intensive care centre for acute myocardial infarction. *Lancet*; **ii**, 349–352.

Bruce R, Blackmon J, Jones J, Strait G (1963) Exercise testing in adult normal subjects and cardiac patients. *Pediatrics*, **32**, 742–756.

Day H (1963) Preliminary studies of an acute coronary care area. *Lancet*; **83**, 53–55.

Detry J, Fox K (1996) Exercise testing. In: Julian D, Camm A, Fox K, *et al.* (eds) *Diseases of the Heart*, 2nd edn. W.B. Saunders, London.

DiMarco J, Philbrick J (1990) Use of ambulatory electrocardiographic (Holter) monitoring. *Annals of Internal Medicine*, **113**, 53–68.

Docherty B (2003) 12 lead ECG interpretation and chest pain management. *British Journal of Nursing*, **12** (21), 1248–1255.

Dower G, Yakush A, Nazzal S, *et al.* (1988) Deriving the 12-lead electrocardiogram from four (EASI) electrodes. *J Electrocardiol*, **21**, S182–S187.

Drew B, Scheinman M (1995) ECG criteria to distinguish between aberrantly conducted supraventricular tachycardia and ventricular tachycardia: practical aspects for the immediate care setting. *Pacing Clin Electrophysio*, **18**, 2194–2208.

Drew B, Adams M (2001) Clinical consequences of ST segment changes caused by body position mimicking transient myocardial ischaemia: hazards of ST-segment monitoring? *Electrocardiol*, **34**, 261–264.

Drew B, Pelter M, Brodnick D, *et al.* (2002) Comparison of a new reduced lead set ECG with the standard ECG for diagnosing cardiac arrhythmias and myocardial ischaemia. *J Etectrocardiol*, **35**, S13–S2l.

Drew B, Califf R, Funk M, *et al.* (2005) AHA Scientific Statement: Practice Standards for Electrocardiographic Monitoring in Hospital Settings. An American Heart Association Scientific Statement from the Councils on Cardiovascular Nursing, Clinical Cardiology, and Cardiovascular Disease in the Young: Endorsed by the International Society of Computerized Electrocardiology and the American Association of Critical-Care Nurses. *Journal of Cardiovascular Nursing*, **20** (2), 76–106.

Falk P, Winnike J, Woodmansee C, *et al.* (2000) Outbreak of vancomycin-resistant enterococci in a burn unit. *Infection Control Hospital & Epidemiology*, **21** (9), 575–582.

Houghton D (2006) ECG equipment: wired for infection? *Nursing*, **36** (12), 71.

Hurst J (1998) Naming of the waves in the ECG, with a brief account of their genesis. *Circulation*, **98**, 1937–1942.

Khan E (2004) Clinical skills: the physiological basis and interpretation of the ECG. *British Journal of Nursing*, **13** (8), 440–446.

Irving J, Bruce R, de Rouen T (1977) Variations in and significance of systolic pressure during maximal exercise (treadmill) testing. *American Journal of Cardiology*, **39**, 841–848.

Jacobson C (2000) Optimum bedside cardiac monitoring. *Progress in Cardiovascular Nursing*, **15** (4), 134–137.

Jancin B (2004) Antibiotic-resistant pathogens found on 77% of EKG lead wires. *Cardiology News*, **2** (3), 14.

Jevon P (2002) *Advanced Cardiac Life Support*. Butterworth Heinemann, Oxford.

Jevon P (2006) Cardiac monitoring part 1; ECG monitoring. *Nursing Times*, **103** (1), 26–27.

Jowett NI, Thompson DR (1995) *Comprehensive Coronary Care*, 2nd edn. Scutari Press, London.

Kennedy H (1992) Importance of the standard electrocardiogram in ambulatory (Holter) electrocardiography. *American Heart Journal*, **123**, 1660–1677.

Knight B, Pelosi F, Michaud G, *et al.* (1999) Clinical consequences of electrocardiographic artifact mimicking ventricular tachycardia. *N Engl J Med*, **341**, 1270–1274.

Khush K, Rapaport E, Waters D (2005) The history of the coronary care unit. *The Canadian Journal of Cardiology*; **21** (12), 1041–1045.

Marriott HJL (1988) *Practical Electrocardiography*, 8th edn. Williams & Wilkins, London.

Mason R, Likar I (1966) A new system of multiple-lead exercise electro-cardiography. *Am Heart J*; **7**, 196–205.

Master A, Friedman R, Dack S (1942) The electrocardiogram after standard exercise as a functional test of the heart. *American Heart Journal*, **24**, 777–793.

Meltzer LE, Pinneo R, Kitchell JR (1983) *Intensive Coronary Care: a Manual for Nurses*, 4th edn. Prentice Hall, London.

Mickley H (1994) Ambulatory ST segment monitoring after myocardial infarction. *British Heart Journal*, **71**, 113–114.

Mirvis DM, Berson AS, Goldberger, AE, *et al.* (1989) Instrumentation and practice standards for electrocardiographic monitoring in special care units: a report for health professionals by a Task Force of the Council on Clinical Cardiology, American Heart Association. *Circulation*, **79**, 464–471.

Naughton J, Ballke B, Nagle F (1964) Refinements in methods of evaluation and physical conditioning before and after myocardial infarction. *American Journal of Cardiology*, **14**, 837–843.

Navas S (2003) Atrial fibrillation: part 1. *Nursing Standard*, **17** (37), 45–54.

Pantridge J (1970) Mobile coronary care. *Chest*, **58**, 229–234.

Pantridge J, Wilson C (1996) A history of pre-hospital coronary care. *Ulster Med J*, **65** (1), 68–73.

Paul S, Hebra J.(1998) *The Nurse's Guide to Cardiac Rhythm Interpretation*. W.B. Saunders, London.

Perez A (1996a) Cardiac monitoring: mastering the essentials. *Registered Nurse*, **59** (8), 32–39.

Petch M (1985) Lessons from ambulatory electrocardiography. *British Medical Journal*, **291**, 617–618.

Quinn T, Thompson D (1999) History and development of coronary care. *Intensive & Critical Care Nursing*, **15** (3), 131–141.

Ren Y, Yang L, Hu P (1998) Analysis of influencing factors on ECG monitoring. *Shanxi Nursing Journal*, **12** (5), 213–214.

Resuscitation Council UK (2006) *Advanced Life Support*, 5th edn. Resuscitation Council UK, London.

Sharman J (2007) Clinical skills: cardiac rhythm recognition and monitoring. *British Journal of Nursing*, **16** (5).

Snellen H (1995) *Willem Einthoven (1860–1927): Father of Electrocardiography*. Kluwer Academic Publishers, Dordrecht, Netherlands.

Soanes C, Stevenson A (2006) *Oxford Dictionary of English*. Oxford University Press, Oxford.

Sykes A, Waller A (1887) The electrocardiogram *BMJ (Clin Res edn)*, **294**, 1396–1398.

Thompson P (1997) *Coronary Care Manual*. Churchill Livingstone, London.

Waller A (1887) A demonstration on man of electromotive changes accompanying the heart's beat. *J Physiol*, **8**, 229–234.

# 3 | ECG Interpretation of Cardiac Arrhythmias

## INTRODUCTION

Cardiac arrhythmia literally means total lack of rhythm. However, any cardiac rhythm that deviates from the normal sinus rhythm, regardless of the rhythm or whether it is due to a disturbance in impulse formation or impulse conduction, can be classified as a cardiac arrhythmia.

Accurate ECG interpretation of cardiac arrhythmias is essential to ensure the most appropriate management. A systematic approach to ECG interpretation of cardiac arrhythmias is therefore paramount.

The aim of this chapter is to understand ECG interpretation of cardiac arrhythmias.

## LEARNING OUTCOMES

At the end of the chapter the reader will be able to:

❑ List the mechanisms of cardiac arrhythmias.
❑ Discuss the classification of cardiac arrhythmias.
❑ Describe a six-stage approach for ECG interpretation of cardiac arrhythmias.

## MECHANISMS OF CARDIAC ARRHYTHMIAS

There are several mechanisms that can lead to cardiac arrhythmias. Each will now be discussed.

### Altered automaticity

Automaticity is the term used to describe the inherent ability of automatic or pacemaker cells to initiate electrical impulses. Altered automaticity can lead to changes in the rate of impulse generation by the SA node, e.g. sinus bradycardia and sinus tachycardia. It is caused by either an increase in autonomic nerve activity or by SA node disease.

If the SA node rate falls or if its impulses are blocked, another group of automatic cells lower down in the conduction system may then take over as pacemaker of the heart, resulting in an escape rhythm.

### Enhanced automaticity

Enhanced automaticity may also cause arrhythmias. Causes of enhanced automaticity include increased sympathetic activity, myocardial ischaemia, digoxin toxicity, drugs, electrolyte imbalances, hyperthermia, hypoxia, hypercapnia and acidosis.

### Re-entry

The re-entry mechanism is the most common cause of clinically significant cardiac arrhythmias, including ventricular fibrillation and most cases of ventricular tachycardia (Tomlin, 1997). The re-entry mechanism is caused by a self-perpetuating 'circus movement' of the cardiac impulse (see Figure 3.1). The re-entry mechanism requires:

- *Non uniform refractoriness*: this can create an area of unidirectional block.
- *Slow conduction*: the conduction time over the re-entry circuit should exceed the longest refractory period of any point in the circuit.

(Julian & Cowan, 1993)

AV nodal re-entrant tachycardia is the commonest cause of paroxysmal regular narrow complex tachycardia (Esberger *et al.*, 2008). AV re-entrant tachycardias can occur owing to the presence of an additional pathway, other than the AV junction, connecting the atria and the ventricles, e.g. bundle of Kent (Wolff-Parkinson-White syndrome). This accessory conduction pathway allows the atrial impulse to bypass the AV junction and activate the ventricles prematurely (ventricular pre-excitation) (Esberger *et al.*, 2008).

### Triggered activity

Triggered activity requires a preceding stimulus to initiate depolarisation – afterdepolarisations are oscillations in the

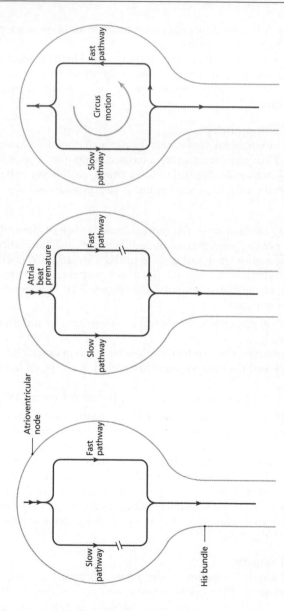

**Figure 3.1** Re-entry causative mechanism of cardiac arrhythmias. Reprinted from Morris F, et al., *ABC of Clinical Electrocardiography*, 2nd edn, copyright 2008, with permission of Blackwell Publishing.

transmembrane potential that are induced by the preceding action potential (Tonkin, 1997). Arrhythmias caused by triggered activity include benign ventricular ectopics, torsades de pointes and ventricular fibrillation (Tonkin, 1997).

### Reperfusion

Reperfusion arrhythmias can occur following spontaneous or drug-induced thrombolysis or coronary angiography (Tonkin, 1997). The duration and severity of ischaemia are thought to be key contributory factors.

There appear to be two distinct time-related mechanisms for reperfusion arrhythmias. Immediately following reperfusion, the 're-entry' mechanism, which can precipitate ventricular fibrillation, is significant. 'Triggered activity' and 'enhanced automaticity' are later mechanisms for reperfusion arrhythmias.

### Conduction disturbances

Conduction disturbances or AV block (slowing down or complete blocking of an impulse) can occur within the AV junction or bundle branches. AV block complicates 10% of myocardial infarctions (Jowett & Thompson, 1995). Conduction disturbances in the AV junction are usually associated with inferior myocardial infarction and those in the bundle branches with anterior myocardial infarction.

### CLASSIFICATION OF CARDIAC ARRHYTHMIAS

Cardiac arrhythmias can be classified into one of two groups: those that result from a disturbance in impulse formation or those that result from a disturbance in impulse conduction (Meltzer et al., 1983) (cardiac arrhythmias are discussed in this book according to this classification).

Although this general classification is helpful, it does have limitations as some arrhythmias may result from a disturbance both in impulse formation and conduction.

### Arrhythmias resulting from a disturbance in impulse formation

Cardiac arrhythmias that result from a disturbance in impulse formation can be categorised according to their site of origin and mechanism of disturbance.

### Site of origin

- *SA node*: sinus rhythms, e.g. sinus bradycardia, sinus arrest.
- *Atria*: atrial rhythms, e.g. atrial ectopics, atrial fibrillation.
- *AV junction*: junctional rhythms, e.g. junction tachycardia.
- *Ventricles*: ventricular rhythms, e.g. ventricular premature beats, ventricular tachycardia.

### Mechanism

- Tachycardia > 100 beats/min.
- Bradycardia < 60 beats/min.
- Premature contractions.
- Flutter.
- Fibrillation.

### Arrhythmias resulting from a disturbance in impulse conduction

Cardiac arrhythmias that result from a disturbance in impulse conduction refer to an abnormal delay or block of the impulse at some point along the conduction system. They are traditionally categorised according to the site of the defect:

- SA node blocks, e.g. SA block.
- AV blocks, e.g. first, second, third degree AV block.
- Intraventricular blocks, e.g. bundle branch blocks.

### SIX-STAGE APPROACH TO ECG INTERPRETATION OF CARDIAC ARRHYTHMIAS

To accurately interpret an ECG trace requires considerable experience and expertise. However, it is possible to interpret most ECG traces and arrive at a reliable diagnosis on which to base effective treatment, by following a systematic approach to ECG interpretation:

- Is electrical activity present?
- What is the QRS rate?
- Is the QRS rhythm regular or irregular?
- Is the QRS complex width normal or broad?
- Are P waves present?
- How are P waves related to QRS complexes?

(Resuscitation Council UK, 2006)

It must be emphasised that displays and ECG printouts from cardiac monitors are suitable for interpreting cardiac arrhythmias only and not for analysis of ST segment changes and more sophisticated ECG interpretation (Resuscitation Council UK, 2006). Wherever possible, a 12 lead ECG should be recorded, as this may provide additional diagnostic information.

The six-stage approach to ECG interpretation of cardiac arrhythmias will now be described.

### Is electrical activity present?

If there is no electrical activity check the gain control (ECG size), ECG leads, ECG electrodes, all electrical connections and the defibrillator/cardiac monitor ensuring it is switched on. If there is still no electrical activity and the patient is pulseless, the diagnosis is asystole (Resuscitation Council UK, 2006). The line is usually distorted due to drift of the baseline, electrical interference and CPR. Sometimes P waves may be present – 'P wave asystole' or ventricular standstill.

A completely straight line is usually caused by disconnection of ECG leads or wrong monitoring lead, e.g. 'paddles' selected on the defibrillator when monitoring with ECG leads. If electrical activity is present, ascertain whether there are any recognisable ECG complexes. If there aren't any, VF is the probable diagnosis. If recognisable ECG complexes can be identified the following five steps should be followed.

### What is the QRS rate?

Estimate the QRS rate by counting the number of large (1 cm) squares between adjacent QRS complexes and dividing it into 300, e.g. the QRS rate in Figure 3.2 is about 85/min (300/3.5). An ECG rate ruler (see Figure 3.3) can also be used.

Care should be taken if the QRS rate is irregular. A more reliable method, if the QRS rate is irregular, is to count the number of QRS complexes in a defined number of seconds and then calculate the rate per minute. For example, if there are 12 QRS complexes in a 10 second strip, then the ventricular rate is 72/min (12 × 6).

The QRS rate can then be classified as:

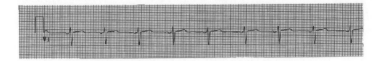

**Figure 3.2** Suggested method for estimating the QRS rate (regular QRS rhythm): divide the number of large squares between two adjacent QRS complexes into 300, i.e. 300/4.2–75/min.

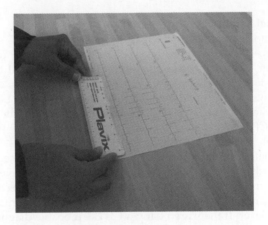

**Figure 3.3** ECG heart rate calculation ruler.

- Normal ventricular rate is 60–100/min
- Bradycardia <60/min
- Tachycardia >100/min

NB A pulse rate of 50 may be 'normal' in some patients and one of 70 may be abnormally slow in other patients.

### Is the QRS rhythm regular or irregular?
Establish whether the QRS rhythm is regular or irregular by carefully comparing the R-R intervals at different sections on the ECG rhythm strip. Callipers may help.

Alternatively, plot two QRS complexes on a piece of paper. Then move the paper to other sections on the rhythm strip and

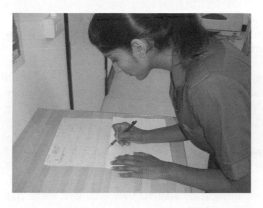

**Figure 3.4** Ascertaining whether the QRS rhythm is regular or irregular.

ascertain whether the marks are aligned exactly with other pairs of QRS complexes (regular QRS rhythm) or not (irregular QRS rhythm) (see Figure 3.4).

If the QRS rhythm is irregular, ascertain whether it is totally irregular, e.g. in atrial fibrillation or whether there is a cyclical pattern to the irregularity, e.g. extrasystoles, pauses, dropped beats, where the relationship between the P waves and QRS complexes is particularly important (see below). The presence of ectopics can render an otherwise regular QRS rhythm irregular. If present, determine whether they are atrial, junctional or ventricular.

### Is the QRS complex width normal or broad?
Note the width of the QRS complex. The normal width is <3 small squares (0.12 seconds). If the width of the QRS complex is broad (3 small squares or more), the rhythm may be ventricular in origin or supraventricular in origin, but transmitted with aberrant conduction. A broad complex tachycardia is most likely to be ventricular in origin.

Examine the QRS complexes and establish whether their morphology is constant. Look to see if ectopics or extrasystoles are present. These can arise from the atria, AV junction and ventricles. By examining their morphology, it is usually possible to determine their origin. If the ectopic QRS complex is narrow (<12 s or 3 small squares), the ectopic focus is situated above the ventricles. If it is wide, the ectopic focus is either above the ventricles, but the impulse is conducted with aberration, or in the ventricles. If they are premature, i.e. before the next anticipated sinus beat, they are commonly termed ectopics. If they are late, i.e. after the next anticipated sinus beat, e.g. following a period of sinus arrest, they are commonly termed escape beats.

### Are P waves present?

Establish whether P waves are present and calculate the rate and regularity. In sinus rhythm the P waves should be identical in shape and upright in lead II. Changes in P wave morphology implies a different pacemaker focus for the impulse. Retrograde activation through the AV junction (junctional or ventricular arrhythmias) usually results in the P waves being inverted in lead II. This is because atrial depolarisation occurs in the opposite direction to normal.

Sometimes it may be difficult to establish whether P waves are present because they are partly or totally obscured by the QRS complexes or T waves, e.g. in sinus tachycardia P waves may merge with the preceding T waves.

In SA block and sinus arrest, P waves will be absent; in atrial fibrillation no P waves can be identified, just a fluctuating baseline, and in atrial flutter, P waves are replaced by regular 'sawtooth' flutter waves, rate approximately 300/min.

### How are P waves related to QRS complexes?

If P waves are present, ascertain whether each one is followed by a QRS complex and whether each QRS complex is preceded by a P wave. Calculate the PR interval; the normal range is 3–5 small squares (0.12–0.20 seconds). A shortened or prolonged PR interval is indicative of a conduction abnormality. Causes of a shortened PR interval include junctional rhythms and impulse conduction via accessory conduction pathways, e.g. bundle of Kent (Wolff-Parkinson-White syndrome). AV block can cause a prolonged PR interval.

If the PR interval is constant it is probable that atrial and ventricular activity is related. If the PR interval is variable establish whether there is a pattern to the variability. Plot out the P waves and QRS complexes and look for any recognisable pattern between the two, the occurrence of missed or dropped beats and PR intervals that vary in a repeated fashion. Complete dissociation between atrial and ventricular activity may be indicative of complete (third degree) atrioventricular heart block.

## CHAPTER SUMMARY
Accurate ECG interpretation of cardiac arrhythmias is essential to ensure the most appropriate management. In this chapter a six-stage approach to ECG interpretation of cardiac arrhythmias has been described.

## REFERENCES
Esberger D, Jones S, Morris F (2008) *ABC of Clinical Electrocardiography*, 2nd edn. Blackwell Publishing, Oxford.

Jowett NI, Thompson DR (1997) *Comprehensive Coronary Care*, 2nd edn. Scutari Press, London.

Julian D, Cowan J (1993) *Cardiology*, 6th edn. Baillière, London.

Meltzer LE, Pinneo R, Kitchell JR (1983) *Intensive Coronary Care: a Manual for Nurses*, 4th edn. Prentice Hall, London.

Resuscitation Council UK (2006) *Advanced Life Support*, 5th edn. Resuscitation Council UK, London.

Tonkin A (1997) Pathophysiology of post infarction ventricular arrhythmias. In: Thompson P (ed.) *Coronary Care Manual*. Churchill Livingstone, London.

# 4 | Cardiac Arrhythmias Originating in the SA Node

## INTRODUCTION

Cardiac arrhythmias originating in the SA node result from a disturbance in impulse formation or impulse conduction within the node itself. The SA node retains its role as pacemaker for the heart, but instead of firing regularly at a rate of 60–100/min, it is firing at a slower, faster or irregular rate. Sometimes the SA node fails to discharge an impulse and activate the atria, either because the impulse is blocked within the node itself or it fails to initiate an impulse.

The aim of this chapter is to recognise cardiac arrhythmias originating in the SA node.

## LEARNING OUTCOMES

At the end of the chapter the reader will be able to discuss the characteristic ECG features, list the causes and outline the treatment of:

❑ Sinus tachycardia.
❑ Sinus bradycardia.
❑ Sinus arrhythmia.
❑ Wandering atrial pacemaker.
❑ SA block.
❑ Sinus arrest.
❑ Sick sinus syndrome.

## SINUS TACHYCARDIA

The term tachycardia derives from the Greek words *takhus* meaning 'swift' and *kardia* meaning 'heart' (Soanes & Stevenson, 2006). Sinus tachycardia can be defined as a sinus rhythm greater than 100 beats/min (Bennett, 2006; Houghton & Gray, 2003). The

ECG has the same characteristics as sinus rhythm, except that the QRS rate is greater than 100 beats/min. The upper limit of sinus tachycardia is usually 140 beats/min (Jowett & Thompson, 1995).

Sinus tachycardia can be a normal response to a physiological stimulus, e.g. exercise, or anxiety. However, if it persists it is usually an indication of pathophysiology (Randall & Ardell, 1990), e.g. shock, pyrexia, heart failure, ischaemic heart disease and pulmonary embolism (Docherty, 2003; Houghton & Gray, 2003). Of particular importance is that it may be a manifestation of heart failure when it is a reflex mechanism to compensate for reduced stroke volume (Meltzer *et al.*, 1983). In myocardial infarction, sinus tachycardia is an adverse prognostic sign (Hjalmarson *et al.*, 1990), because it usually indicates extensive myocardial necrosis associated with excess release of catecholamines (ISIS 2, 1988, Thompson, 1997). Sinus tachycardia at rest is a normal finding in infancy and early childhood (Camm & Katritsis, 1996)

A classical feature which helps distinguish sinus tachycardia from other narrow complex tachycardias, e.g. atrial tachycardia, is that it does not start and end abruptly; both its onset and decline are gradual (Thompson, 1997). Sometimes, in sinus tachycardia, P waves can merge with the preceding QRS complexes. A persistent tachycardia, in the absence of an obvious underlying cause, should prompt careful examination of the ECG: atrial flutter or atrial tachycardia may be the cause of the fast heart rate (Goodacre & Irons, 2008).

## Identifying features on the ECG

- *Electrical activity*: yes.
- *QRS rate*: >100/min, usually ≤140/min.
- *QRS rhythm*: regular.
- *QRS complexes*: normal width and constant morphology.
- *P waves*: present, may be merged into preceding T waves.
- *Relationship between P waves and QRS complexes*: each P wave is followed by a QRS complex and each QRS complex is preceded by a P wave; PR interval is normal and constant.

## Effects on the patient

Most patients with sinus tachycardia are asymptomatic. However, some may complain of palpitations and dyspnoea (Thompson,

1997). As the rate increases, the resultant decreased arterial filling time and reduced stroke volume may lead to a drop in blood pressure and weak peripheral pulses. Sinus tachycardia will increase oxygen consumption and, when associated with myocardial infarction, could extend myocardial necrosis (Jevon, 2002).

### Treatment

Treatment is generally aimed at identifying and, where appropriate, treating the cause. It must be stressed that the intentional slowing down of a sinus tachycardia when it is a normal compensatory mechanism, e.g. in left ventricular failure, can have disastrous consequences on the patient (Houghton & Gray, 2003).

In myocardial infarction, underlying causes should be sought and appropriate treatment instigated promptly (White, 1996). The use of beta-blocking agents, e.g. atenolol, can benefit some patients (ISIS 1, 1986). Sometimes the tachycardia may be pain and/or anxiety induced and may settle with effective pain relief. Any electrolyte imbalances should be corrected. Rarely, catheter ablation therapy on the sinus node is undertaken if drugs have failed to control the rate (Davis 1997).

### Interpretation of Figure 4.1

- *Electrical activity*: present.
- *QRS rate*: 115/min.
- *QRS rhythm*: regular.
- *QRS width*: normal width and constant morphology; ST elevation is present.
- *P waves*: present, constant morphology.
- *Relationship between P waves and QRS complexes*: each P wave is followed by a QRS complex and each QRS complex is preceded by a P wave; PR interval is normal and constant.

The ECG in Figure 4.1 displays sinus tachycardia. This patient was admitted to CCU with an acute inferior myocardial infarction (the ST elevation is suggestive of myocardial damage; a 12 lead ECG helped to confirm this diagnosis). He was complaining of severe central chest pain and was very anxious.

Sinus tachycardia, and not bradycardia, is an unusual clinical finding in an inferior myocardial infarction and it was important to try to identify the underlying cause. Possible causes included patient anxiety, chest pain, heart failure and cardiogenic shock. Following diamorphine 5 mg administered IV, the patient's pain eased and he settled. The heart rate gradually slowed down to 65 beats/min. Chest pain and anxiety were the most probable underlying causes of the sinus tachycardia. There was no clinical evidence of a low cardiac output. The patient's blood pressure and respiratory rate were within normal limits.

### Interpretation of Figure 4.2

- *Electrical activity*: present.
- *QRS rate*: 150/min.
- *QRS rhythm*: regular.
- *QRS*: normal width and constant morphology.
- *P waves*: present and constant morphology.
- *Relationship between P waves and QRS complexes*: each P wave is followed by a QRS complex and each QRS complex is preceded by a P wave; PR interval is normal and constant.

This patient was referred by his general practitioner with a sudden onset of dyspnoea. The ECG displays sinus tachycardia with a ventricular rate of 150/min. BP was 90/60, respiratory rate was 34/min and the patient was pale, cold and clammy. He was also orthopnoeic and expectorating frothy bloodstained sputum. Chest auscultation confirmed the presence of widespread respiratory crackles: left ventricular failure and pulmonary oedema were the cause.

It is likely that the sinus tachycardia was secondary to acute left ventricular failure. Following effective treatment of the primary problem with oxygen, diuretics, nitrates and a small dose of diamorphine, the patient settled and the tachycardia gradually slowed (a characteristic sign of sinus tachycardia).

This is an unusually rapid rate for sinus tachycardia. A tachycardia of this rate could have been caused by an atrial tachyarrhythmia, e.g. atrial tachycardia. However, the PR interval is normal, not short. Close inspection of the 12 lead ECG did confirm sinus tachycardia.

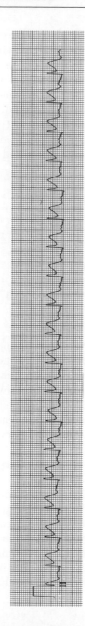

**Figure 4.1** Sinus tachycardia.

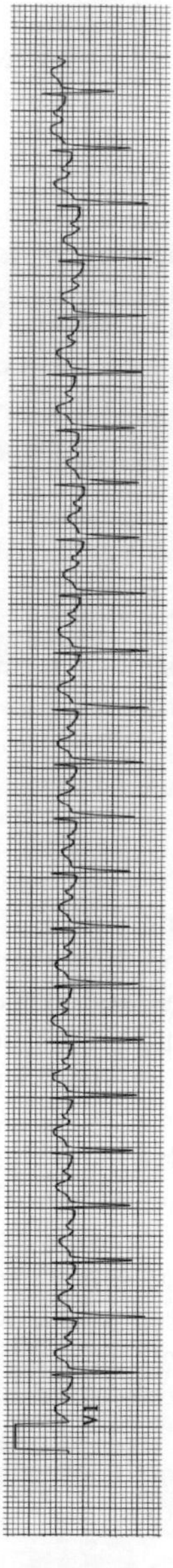

**Figure 4.2** Sinus tachycardia.

### Interpretation of Figure 4.3

- *Electrical activity*: present.
- *QRS rate*: 150/min.
- *QRS rhythm*: regular.
- *QRS*: normal width and constant morphology.
- *P waves*: present and constant morphology.
- *Relationship between P waves and QRS complexes*: each P wave is followed by a QRS complex and each QRS complex is preceded by a P wave; PR interval is normal and constant.

This patient was undergoing a dobutamine stress test (prior to Myoview Perfusion Scan). The extreme tachycardia was actually the desired result of the stress test. The patient, however, was starting to develop chest pain and the stress test had to be stopped.

### Interpretation of Figure 4.4

- *Electrical activity*: present
- *QRS rate*: 130/min.
- *QRS rhythm*: regular
- *QRS*: normal width and constant morphology.
- *P waves*: present and constant morphology.
- *Relationship between P waves and QRS complexes*: each P wave is followed by a QRS complex and each QRS complex is preceded by a P wave; PR interval is normal and constant.

This 24-year-old lady was admitted with a pyrexia and non-blanching rash. She was subsequently diagnosed with endocarditis. She developed an abscess which encroached on the bundle of His, resulting in first degree AV block (see pages 135–137). She was started on antibiotics.

### SINUS BRADYCARDIA

The term bradycardia derives from the Greek words *bradus* meaning 'slow' and *kardia* meaning 'heart' (Soanes & Stevenson, 2006). Sinus bradycardia can be defined as a sinus rhythm of less than 60/min (Bennett, 2006; Da Costa *et al.*, 2008); the ECG has the same characteristics as sinus rhythm, except that the QRS rate is less than 60/min.

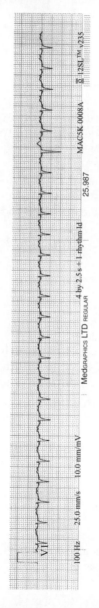

**Figure 4.3** Sinus tachycardia.

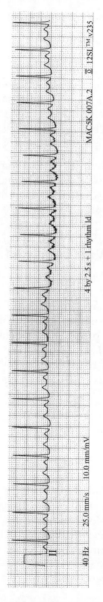

**Figure 4.4** Sinus tachycardia.

The commonest cause of sinus bradycardia is physiological. It can occur in acute myocardial infarction (MI), particularly inferior myocardial infarction (Adgey *et al.*, 1971), because the inferior myocardial wall, the SA node and the AV node are all usually supplied by the right coronary artery (Da Costa *et al.*, 2008). Other causes include certain medical conditions such as hypothermia (Resuscitation Council UK, 2006) and hypothyroidism (Vanhaelst & Neve, 1967), vagal stimulation, e.g. during tracheal suction, increased intracranial pressure, hypoxia, severe pain, hypothermia and drugs such as beta blockers. It can be a normal clinical finding in some patients, e.g. athletes.

Sinus bradycardia may also be caused by sinus node dysfunction (Levy & Mogensen, 1996). Conditions associated with sinus node dysfunction include age, ischaemia, high vagal tone, myocarditis and digoxin toxicity (Da Costa *et al.*, 2008).

### Identifying features on the ECG

- *Electrical activity*: present.
- *QRS rate*: ≤60/min.
- *QRS rhythm*: regular.
- *QRS width*: normal width and constant morphology.
- *P waves*: present, constant morphology.
- *Relationship between P waves and QRS complexes*: P wave is followed by a QRS complex and each QRS complex is preceded by a P wave; PR interval is normal and constant.

### Effects on the patient

Many patients are able to tolerate heart rates of 40/min surprisingly well (Da Costa *et al.*, 2008). Some patients are asymptomatic. It can be a normal physiological state in fit people, e.g. athletes. It may be the desired effect of beta-blocker drug administration. It is common in the early stages of inferior myocardial infarction, rarely requiring treatment (Nolan *et al.*, 1998).

However, the patient may be symptomatic, particularly if the bradycardia is of a sudden onset or is <40/min (Resuscitation Council UK, 2006). Adverse signs include hypotension, chest pain, lightheadedness, dizziness, nausea, syncope, and pale, clammy skin (Da Costa *et al.*, 2008). In addition, escape rhythms are more likely to occur which can predispose to ventricular tachyarrhythmias (Jowett & Thompson, 1995).

## Treatment

Treatment is indicated only if adverse signs (see pages 221–22 and 224) are present and/or there is a risk of asystole (Resuscitation Council UK, 2006). If necessary, oxygen should be administered and IV access secured. If treatment is required, atropine 500 mcg should be administered IV and the ECG rhythm reassessed. Further doses may be required. Cardiac pacing may be required in some situations. The possible cause of the bradycardia should be established, as attention to this (e.g. omitting medication) may provide the most effective treatment. Any electrolyte imbalances should be corrected. Expert help may be required. For further information on the treatment of sinus bradycardia see pages 222 and 224–25.

## Interpretation of Figure 4.5

- *Electrical activity*: present.
- *QRS rate*: 42/min.
- *QRS rhythm*: regular.
- *QRS width*: normal width and constant morphology.
- *P waves*: present and constant morphology.
- *Relationship between P waves and QRS complexes*: each P wave is followed by a QRS complex and each QRS complex is preceded by a P wave; PR interval normal and constant.

The ECG in Figure 4.5 displays sinus bradycardia. The ECG has the same characteristics as sinus rhythm except that the QRS rate is <60 beats/min. This patient had been admitted with an acute inferior myocardial infarction.

In myocardial infarction, bradycardia reduces myocardial oxygen requirements and, as long as the patient remains asymptomatic, no treatment is required (White, 1996). The patient did not present with any adverse signs (see pages 221–22 and 224) and he was not taking any medications prior to admission that could cause a bradycardia (e.g. a beta blocker). The blood pressure was stable, the bradycardia transient and no treatment was required specifically for the bradycardia, though reperfusion therapy was indicated. Subsequently, the patient was closely monitored during the period of bradycardia in order to detect the occurrence of adverse signs.

## Interpretation of Figure 4.6

- *Electrical activity*: present.
- *QRS rate*: 26/min.
- *QRS rhythm*: regular.
- *QRS width*: very broad (0.16 s or 4 small squares) and constant morphology.
- *P waves*: present and constant morphology.
- *Relationship between P waves and QRS complexes*: each P wave is followed by a QRS complex and each QRS complex is preceded by a P wave; PR interval normal and constant.

The ECG in Figure 4.6 displays profound sinus bradycardia. The ECG has the same characteristics as sinus rhythm except that the QRS rate is <60 beats/min. In addition, the QRS complex is very wide, suggestive of bundle branch block (a 12 lead ECG confirmed left bundle branch block).

This patient had been admitted with an acute anterior myocardial infarction. The patient was assessed for the presence of adverse signs (see pages 221–22 and 224). BP was 75/40 and the patient was semi-conscious. He was also very pale and clammy, though these signs are often associated with acute myocardial infarction.

It was quickly established that the patient was severely haemodynamically compromised and urgent intervention to treat the bradycardia was required. The patient was placed in a supine position and oxygen was administered. Atropine 500 mcg was administered IV and then the patient was reassessed. Despite further doses of atropine, the bradycardia did not respond and the patient remained compromised. External pacing, quickly followed by transvenous pacing, was required. This patient subsequently required a permanent pacemaker.

## Interpretation of Figure 4.7

- *Electrical activity*: present.
- *QRS rate*: 42/min.
- *QRS rhythm*: regular.

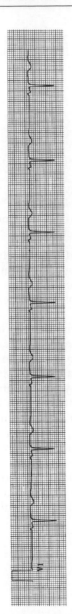

**Figure 4.5** Sinus bradycardia.

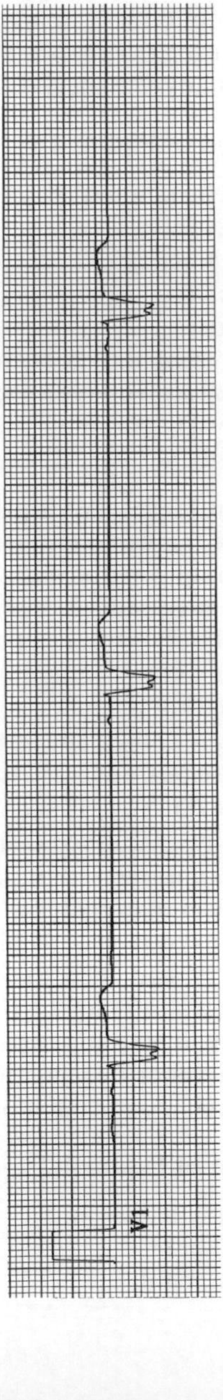

**Figure 4.6** Sinus bradycardia.

- *QRS width*: very broad (0.16 s or 4 small squares) and constant morphology.
- *P waves*: present and constant morphology.
- *Relationship between P waves and QRS complexes*: each P wave is followed by a QRS complex and each QRS complex is preceded by a P wave; PR interval normal and constant.

The ECG in Figure 4.7 displays sinus bradycardia. This patient presented for a dobutamine stress test. He was taking bisoprolol, a beta blocker. Due to the quite marked bradycardia, although the patient was not compromised and had no ill effects, the cardiologist reduced the dose of bisoprolol.

## SINUS ARRHYTHMIA

Sinus arrhythmia is a variation of sinus rhythm characterised by alternate periods of slow and more rapid sinus node discharge (Reynolds, 1996; Bennett, 2006). The ECG characteristics are identical to sinus rhythm, except that the QRS rhythm is slightly irregular. It is a normal finding and is usually associated with the phases of respiration, increasing with inspiration and decreasing with expiration. The 'beat to beat' variation in the R–R interval is due to a vagally mediated response to increased venous return to the heart during inspiration (Meek & Morris, 2008).

It is a common finding in young persons (Bennett, 2006), but is rarely seen in persons over the age of 40 years (Houghton & Gray, 2003). Sometimes sinus arrhythmia is associated with ischaemia or digoxin toxicity (Reynolds, 1996). In addition, the irregular QRS rhythm can be mistaken for other arrhythmias, e.g. atrial fibrillation.

### Identifying features on the ECG

- *Electrical activity*: present.
- *QRS rate*: 60–100/min.
- *QRS rhythm*: slightly irregular.
- *QRS width*: normal and constant morphology.
- *P waves*: present and constant morphology.
- *Relationship between P waves and QRS complexes*: each P wave is followed by a QRS complex and each QRS complex is preceded by a P wave; PR interval normal and constant.

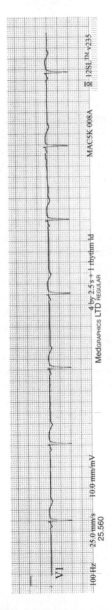

**Figure 4.7** Sinus bradycardia.

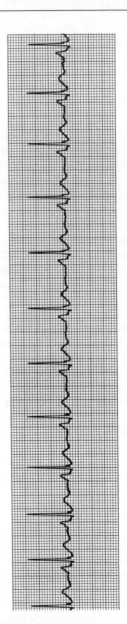

**Figure 4.8** Sinus arrhythmia.

**Effects on the patient**

No ill effects reported.

**Treatment**

It is harmless; no treatment or investigations are necessary (Houghton & Gray, 2003).

**Interpretation of Figure 4.8**

- *Electrical activity*: present.
- *QRS rate*: 75/min.
- *QRS rhythm*: slightly irregular.
- *QRS width*: normal and constant morphology.
- *P waves*: present and constant morphology.
- *Relationship between P waves and QRS complexes*: each P wave is followed by a QRS complex and each QRS complex is preceded by a P wave; PR interval normal and constant.

The ECG in Figure 4.8 displays sinus arrhythmia. Close inspection confirmed that the irregularity of the rhythm was not a serious arrhythmia, e.g. atrial fibrillation. This ECG strip was recorded in a 37-year-old male. The heart rate fluctuated with respiration.

**Interpretation of Figure 4.9**

- *Electrical activity*: present.
- *QRS rate*: 75/min.
- *QRS rhythm*: regularly/irregular
- *QRS width*: 120 ms (right bundle branch block pattern) and constant morphology.
- *P waves*: present and constant morphology
- *Relationship between P waves and QRS complexes*: each P wave is followed by a QRS complex and each QRS complex is preceded by a P wave; PR interval normal and constant.

The ECG in Figure 4.9 displays profound sinus arrhythmia. This EGC was recorded in a 63-year-old gentleman who was hyperventilating. The heart rate fluctuated with respiration.

## WANDERING ATRIAL PACEMAKER

A wandering atrial pacemaker is characterised by the pacemaker 'wandering' from the SA node down to the atria or AV junction. It is usually related to vagal influences (Meltzer *et al.*, 1983). It can occur in healthy young people, but it may be a manifestation of atrial pathology (Thompson, 1997).

### Identifying features on the ECG

- *Electrical activity*: present.
- *QRS rate*: usually normal.
- *QRS rhythm*: regular.
- *QRS width*: normal width and constant morphology.
- *P waves*: present, morphology and position will vary depending on the site of origin of the impulse.
- *Relationship between P waves and QRS complexes*: each P wave is followed by a QRS complex and each QRS complex is preceded by a P wave; PR interval may vary depending on the site of the origin of the impulse.

### Effects on the patient

There are no effects on the patient.

### Treatment

No treatment required. Any electrolyte imbalances should be corrected.

## SA BLOCK

In SA block the impulse from the node itself is blocked and fails to transverse the junction between the SA node and the surrounding atrial myocardium (Bennett, 2006). This results in a dropped beat. Just as with AV junctional block, SA block can be classified as first, second and third degree block.

However, only second degree SA block can be diagnosed from the ECG. Intermittent failure of atrial activation results in PP intervals which are multiples (usually twice) of the cycle length during sinus rhythm (Bennett, 1994). On the ECG a complete PQRST complex is absent, but the next sinus beat arises at the expected time. Causes of SA block include idiopathic fibrosis of the SA node, cardiomyopathy, myocardial ischaemia/infarction.

### Identifying features on the ECG

- *Electrical activity*: present.
- *QRS rate*: usually normal, sometimes <60/min.
- *QRS rhythm*: dropped beats results in an irregular rhythm.
- *QRS width*: normal width and constant morphology.
- *P waves*: absent during period of SA block, otherwise present and constant morphology.
- *Relationship between P waves and QRS complexes*: PQRST complex absent during period of SA block, otherwise each P wave is followed by a QRS complex and each QRS complex is preceded by a P wave; PR interval normal and constant.

### Effects on the patient

This rarely affects the patient, although syncope may occur if pauses are prolonged or occur frequently.

### Treatment

SA block is of little clinical importance, except that it may be a manifestation of toxicity with digoxin or other anti-arrhythmic drugs (Julian & Cowan, 1993). Dose reduction or withdrawal of drug(s) that the patient is taking may be required. Any electrolyte imbalances should be corrected.

### Interpretation of Figure 4.10

- *Electrical activity*: present.
- *QRS rate*: approximately 60–70/min.
- *QRS rhythm*: dropped beats results in an irregular rhythm.
- *QRS width*: normal width and constant morphology, one dropped beat.
- *P waves*: absent during period of SA block, otherwise present and constant morphology; PP intervals are constant despite the dropped beat – this is suggestive of SA block.
- *Relationship between P waves and QRS complexes*: PQRST complex absent during period of SA block, otherwise each P wave is followed by a QRS complex and each QRS complex is preceded by a P wave; PR interval normal and constant.

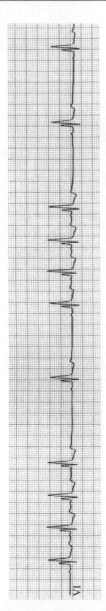

**Figure 4.9** Sinus arrhythmia.

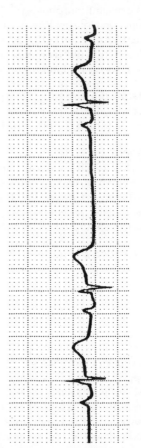

**Figure 4.10** SA block.

The ECG in Figure 4.10 displays second degree SA block. The patient did not display any adverse signs and there were no episodes of syncope. The patient had been taking digoxin (125 mcg once daily) for several years for 'atrial fibrillation'. As the ECG trace displays, the patient was no longer in atrial fibrillation, and because the arrhythmia could have been caused by digoxin, the drug was stopped while the patient's digoxin levels were measured.

## SINUS ARREST

Sinus arrest is when the SA node fails to initiate an impulse. It is characterised by absent P waves and cardiac standstill for varying periods of time, with escape beats from the atria, AV junction or ventricles usually taking over pacemaker function (escape rhythm) (Jowett & Thompson, 1995).

Causes of sinus arrest include idiopathic fibrosis of the SA node, cardiomyopathy and myocardial ischaemia/infarction. Intermittent sinus arrest may occur following an inferior myocardial infarction.

### Identifying features on the ECG

- *Electrical activity*: present.
- *QRS rate*: normal or <60/min.
- *QRS rhythm*: irregular due to dropped beats.
- *QRS width*: usually normal width and constant morphology; if escape beats present these may be of different morphology depending on their site of origin.
- *P waves*: absent during period of SA block, otherwise present and constant morphology.
- *Relationship between P waves and QRS complexes*: PQRST complex absent during period of sinus arrest, otherwise each P wave is followed by a QRS complex and each QRS complex is preceded by a P wave; PR interval normal and constant.

### Effects on the patient

Although the haemodynamic effect on the patient is usually self-limiting owing to the junctional or ventricular escape beats maintaining a cardiac output, it may still be severe enough to cause syncope (Thompson, 1997).

**Treatment**

Atropine will be required during periods of sinus arrest if adverse signs (see pages 221–22 and 224) are present (Resuscitation Council UK, 2006). If recurrent and causing syncope, a permanent pacemaker may be required (Thompson, 1997). Any electrolyte imbalances should be corrected.

**Interpretation of Figure 4.11**

- *Electrical activity*: present.
- *QRS rate*: difficult to determine (longer ECG strip required).
- *QRS rhythm*: irregular, 4.5 s pause present.
- *QRS width*: normal width and constant morphology.
- *P waves*: absent during sinus arrest, otherwise present and constant morphology.
- *Relationship between P waves and QRS complexes*: absent QRS complexes owing to sinus arrest and no escape rhythms present; otherwise each P wave is followed by a QRS complex and each QRS complex is preceded by a P wave; PR interval normal and constant.

The ECG in Figure 4.11 displays sinus arrest. Profound adverse signs were present. BP was unrecordable and the patient was cold, pale, clammy, semi-conscious and agitated.

It was quickly established that the patient was severely haemo-dynamically compromised and urgent intervention to treat the sinus arrest and the resultant bradycardia was required. The patient was placed in a supine position and oxygen administered. Atropine 500 mcg was administered IV and the patient reassessed. After a second dose of atropine, the heart rate improved. The sinus arrest was transient and the cause was thought to be inferior myocardial ischaemia. No further treatment for the arrhythmia was required.

## SICK SINUS SYNDROME

Sick sinus syndrome is the term used to describe a condition that encompasses a variety of cardiac arrhythmias related to abnormal

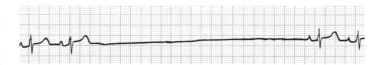

**Figure 4.11** Sinus arrest.

SA node and atrial activity (Ferrer, 1973). A common cause of syncope, dizzy episodes and palpitations, sick sinus syndrome is more common in the elderly although it may occur at any age (Bennett, 2006).

Sick sinus syndrome can be classified as follows:

- Intermittent sinus arrest.
- Stable sinus bradycardia.
- Tachycardia-bradycardia ('tachy-brady') syndrome – the tachycardia is usually atrial fibrillation

(Thompson, 1997)

The exact cause of sick sinus syndrome is unknown, although histologic degeneration of the SA node, AV junction and the conduction tissues between the two is often found on post-mortem (Ornato & Peberdy, 1996).

### Identifying features on the ECG

Identifying features will depend on the arrhythmias (see above).

### Effects on the patient

The patient may complain of palpitations if tachyarrhythmic episodes present. During periods of severe bradycardia or asystole the patient may experience a syncope attack.

### Treatment

Patients with persistent symptomatic bradycardia usually require permanent ventricular or AV sequential pacing (Ornato & Peberdy, 1996). Patients with the tachy-brady syndrome may also require concurrent anti-arrhythmic therapy. However, with the increasing use of dual chamber pacemakers, sick sinus syndrome can often be controlled with just pacemaker therapy (Thompson, 1997). Any electrolyte imbalances should be corrected.

## CHAPTER SUMMARY
Cardiac arrhythmias originating in the SA node result from a disturbance in impulse formation or impulse conduction within the node itself. The SA node usually retains its role as pacemaker for the heart, but instead of firing regularly at a rate of 60–100/min, it is firing at a slower (sinus bradycardia), faster (sinus tachycardia) or irregular (sinus arrhythmia) rate. Sometimes the SA node fails to discharge an impulse and activate the atria, either because the impulse is blocked (SA block) within the node itself or because it fails to initiate an impulse (sinus arrest).

## REFERENCES
Adgey A, Geddes J, Webb S, *et al.* (1971) Acute phase of myocardial infarction. *Lancet*, **2**, 501–504.

Bennett DH (1994) *Cardiac Arrhythmias*, 4th edn. Butterworth Heinemann, Oxford.

Bennett DH (2006) *Cardiac Arrhythmias*, 6th edn. Butterworth Heinemann, Oxford.

Camm A, Katritsis D (1996) The diagnosis of tachyarrhythmias. In: Julian D, Camm AJ, Fox KM, *et al.* (eds) *Diseases of the Heart*, 2nd edn. W.B. Saunders, London.

Da Costa D, Brady W, Redhouse J (2008) Bradycardias and atrioventricular conduction block. In: Morris F, Brady W, Camm J (eds) *ABC of Clinical Electrocardiography*, 2nd edn. Blackwell Publishing, Oxford.

Davis M (1997) Catheter ablation therapy of arrhythmias. In: Thompson P (ed.) *Coronary Care Manual*. Churchill Livingstone, London.

Docherty B (2003) 12 lead ECG interpretation and chest pain management. *British Journal of Nursing*, **12** (21), 1248–1255.

Ferrer M (1973) The sick sinus syndrome. *Circulation*, **47**, 635–641.

Goodacre S, Irons R (2008) Atrial arrhythmias. In: Morris F, Brady W, Camm J (eds) *ABC of Clinical Electrocardiography*, 2nd edn. Blackwell Publishing, Oxford.

Hjalmarson A, Gilpin E, Kjekshus J, *et al.* (1990) Influence of heart rate on mortality after myocardial infarction. *American Journal of Cardiology*, **65**, 547–553.

Houghton A, Gray D (2003) *Making Sense of the ECG: a Hands-on Guide*, 2nd edn. Hodder-Arnold, London.

ISIS 1 (First International Study of Infarct Survival) (1986) Collaborative Group. A randomised trail of intravenous atenolol among 16027 cases of suspected myocardial infarction. *Lancet*, **2**, 57–66.

ISIS 2 (1988) Collaborative Group. A randomised trial of intravenous streptokinase, oral aspirin, both, or neither among 17187 cases of suspected acute myocardial infarction. *Lancet*, **2**, 349.

Jevon P (2002) *Advanced Cardiac Life Support*. Butterworth Heinemann, Oxford.

Jowett NI, Thompson DR (1995) *Comprehensive Coronary Care*, 2nd edn. Scutari Press, London.

Julian D, Cowan J (1993) *Cardiology*, 6th edn. Baillière, London.

Levy S, Mogensen L (1996) Diagnosis of bradycardias. In: Julian D, Camm AJ, Fox KM, *et al.* (eds) *Diseases of the Heart*, 2nd edn. W.B. Saunders, London.

Meek S, Morris F (2008) Introduction. 1-leads, rate, rhythm and cardiac axis. In: Morris F, Brady W, Camm J (eds) *ABC of Clinical Electrocardiography*, 2nd edn. Blackwell Publishing, Oxford.

Meltzer LE, Pinneo R, Kitchell JR (1983) *Intensive Coronary Care: a Manual for Nurses*, 4th edn. Prentice Hall, London.

Nolan J, Greenwood J, Mackintosh A (1998) *Cardiac Emergencies: a Pocket Guide*. Butterworth Heinemann, Oxford.

Ornato J, Peberdy M (1996) Etiology, electrophysiology, and myocardial mechanics of bradyasystolic states. In: Paradis N, Halperin H, Nowak R (eds) *Cardiac Arrest: the Science and Practice of Resuscitation Medicine*. Williams & Wilkins, London.

Randall W, Ardell J (1990) Nervous control of the heart: anatomy and pathophysiology. In: Zipes D, Jalife J (eds) *Cardiac Electrophysiology: From Cell to Bedside*. W.B. Saunders, Philadelphia.

Resuscitation Council UK (2006) *Advanced Life Support*, 5th edn. Resuscitation Council UK, London.

Reynolds G (1996) The resting electrocardiogram. In: Julian D, Camm AJ, Fox KM, *et al.* (eds) *Diseases of the Heart*, 2nd edn. W.B. Saunders, London.

Soanes C, Stevenson A (2006) *Oxford Dictionary of English*. Oxford University Press, Oxford.

Thompson P (1997) *Coronary Care Manual*. Churchill Livingstone, London.

Vanhaelst I, Neve P (1967) Coronary artery disease and hypothyroidism. *Lancet*, **2**, 800.

White H (1996) Myocardial infarction. In: Julian D, Camm AJ, Fox KM, *et al.* (eds) *Diseases of the Heart*, 2nd edn. W.B. Saunders, London.

# 5 | Cardiac Arrhythmias Originating in the Atria

## INTRODUCTION

Cardiac arrhythmias originating in the atria result primarily from either ischaemic damage to, or over distension of, the atrial walls. If P waves are present they are usually of different morphology from sinus P waves. As the ventricles are activated via the normal conduction pathways, the QRS complex is usually narrow and of a normal morphology. Any complications resulting from atrial arrhythmias are usually associated with the tachycardic rate and/or loss of effective atrial contractions (atrial kick), resulting in a fall in cardiac output of 20–30% (Stewart, 2002).

The aim of this chapter is to be able to recognise cardiac arrhythmias originating in the atria.

## LEARNING OUTCOMES

At the end of the chapter the reader will be able to discuss the characteristic ECG features, list the causes and outline the treatment of:

❑ Atrial ectopic beats.
❑ Atrial tachycardia.
❑ Atrial flutter.
❑ Atrial fibrillation.

## ATRIAL ECTOPIC BEATS

The term ectopic can literally be defined as an abnormal place or position (the term originates from the Greek word *ektopos* meaning 'out of place' (Soanes & Stevenson, 2006). The terms ectopic beat, premature beat (APBs) and extrasystole are synonymous (Bennett, 2006; Houghton & Gray, 2003). The term ectopic is preferred by the Resuscitation Council UK (2006) and will be used in this book.

Atrial ectopics are caused by a focus in the atria (and very occasionally in the SA node itself) (Camm & Katritsis, 1996), firing earlier in the cardiac cycle than the next timed beat would be expected (Bennett, 2006). They are common (Docherty, 2003). They can be a normal finding and can be worsened by cardiac stimulants, e.g. tobacco, caffeine and alcohol (Thompson, 1997). They can occur in patients with chronic obstructive pulmonary disease (CPOD), particularly those with an acute respiratory tract infection, respiratory failure or pulmonary embolism (Harrigan & Jones, 2008). They can complicate heart disease, especially atrial enlargement, and may herald the onset of atrial fibrillation, atrial flutter or atrial tachycardia.

Atrial ectopics occur prior to the next anticipated sinus beat (Camm & Katritsis, 1996), i.e. the P wave will be premature. As the site of origin of the P wave and the direction of atrial depolarisation will differ to that during sinus rhythm, the resultant P wave will have a different shape (morphology) to the P wave of sinus rhythm (Bennett, 2006). The QRS complex is usually identical to the one during sinus rhythm because the ventricles are usually depolarised in the normal way (Docherty, 2003). The ensuing pause is approximately equal to or marginally longer than the normal sinus RR interval. The pause is caused by the atrial ectopic depressing SA node automaticity (Bennett, 2006).

Sometimes, an atrial ectopic is not conducted to the ventricles because it has arisen so early in the cardiac cycle that the AV junction is still refractory and unable to conduct it. This is a common cause of unexpected pauses (Camm & Katritsis, 1996). Atrial bigeminy is when an atrial ectopic occurs every second beat and atrial trigeminy is when one occurs every third beat (Marriott, 1988).

### Identifying features on the ECG

- *Electrical activity*: present.
- *QRS rate*: usually normal, though dependent upon underlying rhythm and frequency of APBs.
- *QRS rhythm*: slightly irregular owing to presence of APBs.
- *QRS width*: usually normal width and constant morphology; the prematurity of the APB may result in the impulse being

conducted to the ventricles with bundle branch block – QRS morphology will then differ.

- *P waves*: present; those associated with APBs will be of different morphology from sinus P waves and may be superimposed on the preceding T waves.
- *Relationship between P waves and QRS complexes*: each P wave is followed by a QRS complex and each QRS complex is preceded by a P wave; PR interval may be marginally longer than in sinus rhythm (Camm & Katritsis, 1996).

**Effects on the patient**

The most common symptom is palpitation; the patient is usually aware of the premature contraction itself, not of the following pause often described as a 'missed beat' or of a stronger post-ectopic beat (Camm & Katritsis, 1996). The palpitations are more evident at night when the patient is in a left lateral position, during or immediately following exercise and while sitting quietly (Camm & Katritsis 1996). On rare occasions the patient may experience chest pain. The patient may be asymptomatic.

**Treatment**

Atrial ectopics are benign and no treatment is necessary. Any electrolyte imbalances should be corrected.

**Interpretation of Figure 5.1**

- *Electrical activity*: present.
- *QRS rate*: 75/min.
- *QRS rhythm*: slightly irregular owing to APB.
- *QRS widths*: normal width and constant morphology.
- *P waves*: present; the P wave associated with the atrial ectopic is of different morphology from the sinus P waves.
- *Relationship between P waves and QRS complexes*: each P wave is followed by a QRS complex and each QRS complex is preceded by a P wave; the PR interval associated with the atrial ectopic is shorter than the PR interval in the sinus beats.

The ECG in Figure 5.1 displays sinus rhythm with an atrial ectopic. This patient was admitted to the ward with increasing episodes of chest pain. When checking her pulse, it was found to be slightly irregular. Cardiac monitoring confirmed that this was due to the presence of occasional APBs. No treatment was required. In fact, a few hours after admission the atrial ectopics ceased occurring, thus suggesting their likely underlying cause was patient anxiety.

## Interpretation of Figure 5.2

- *Electrical activity*: present.
- *QRS rate*: 95/min.
- *QRS rhythm*: slightly irregular owing to presence of atrial ectopics.
- *QRS width*: normal width and constant morphology.
- *P waves*: present, those associated with the atrial ectopics are superimposed on the preceding T waves – not possible to assess their morphology.
- *Relationship between P waves and QRS complexes*: each P wave is followed by a QRS complex and each QRS complex is preceded by a P wave; PR interval associated with the atrial ectopics is difficult to calculate.

The ECG in Figure 5.2 displays sinus rhythm with atrial ectopics. This patient was admitted to the ward with a history of palpitations and thyrotoxicosis. There were no adverse signs present. However, the patient was commenced on cardiac monitoring because the frequency of atrial ectopics together with a diagnosis of thyrotoxicosis increased the probability of atrial arrhythmias, particularly atrial fibrillation.

## Interpretation of Figure 5.3

- *Electrical activity*: present.
- *QRS rate*: approximately 50/min.
- *QRS rhythm*: slightly irregular owing to presence of atrial ectopic.
- *QRS width*: normal width and constant morphology.
- *P waves*: present; one atrial ectopic has occurred very early in the cardiac cycle.
- *Relationship between P waves and QRS complexes*: except for one P wave (atrial ectopic), each P wave is followed by a QRS

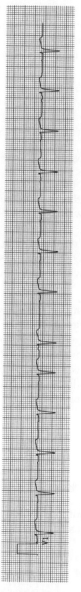

**Figure 5.1** Atrial premature beat.

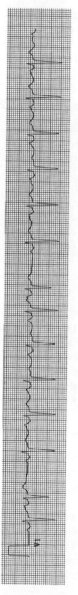

**Figure 5.2** Frequent atrial premature beats use.

complex and each QRS complex is preceded by a P wave; PR interval constant.

The ECG in Figure 5.3 displays a non-conducted atrial ectopic, resulting in a pause. The atrial ectopic has not been conducted to the ventricles because it has arisen so early in the cycle that the AV junction is still refractory and unable to conduct it. This was only an isolated non-conducted atrial ectopic and no treatment was required.

## ATRIAL TACHYCARDIA

Atrial tachycardia is caused by an ectopic focus in the atria rapidly depolarising and overriding the normal pacemaker function of the SA node. It is often preceded by premature atrial contractions and is characterised by a sudden onset and an abrupt end (Meltzer *et al.*, 1983). The atrial rate is normally between 150 and 250/min (Goodacre & Irons, 2008). Although the AV junction may conduct all the impulses, there is often a degree of AV block (Bennett, 2006), particularly if there is associated digoxin toxicity.

Causes of atrial tachycardia include cardiomyopathy, sick sinus syndrome, ischaemic heart disease and rheumatic heart disease (Houghton & Gray, 2003). Multifocal atrial tachycardia can occur in critically ill elderly patients with respiratory disease. It is characterised by multiple atrial foci resulting in P waves of varying morphology and of a variable rate (Goodacre & Irons, 2008).

Carotid sinus massage is often helpful with diagnosis (Bennett, 2006). It produces a transient increase in AV block with a corresponding drop in the ventricular rate (Julian & Cowan, 1993). Adenosine may also aid diagnosis (Goodacre & Irons, 2008). Sometimes it can be difficult to distinguish sinus tachycardia and atrial tachycardia, the P-R interval is usually short in the former and long in the latter (Bennett, 2006).

### Identifying features on the ECG

- *Electrical activity*: present.
- *QRS rate*: usually 150–200/min.

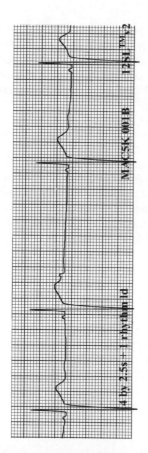

**Figure 5.3** Non-conducted atrial premature beat.

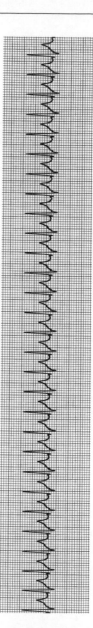

**Figure 5.4** Atrial tachycardia.

- *QRS rhythm*: regular.
- *QRS width*: normal width and morphology.
- *P waves*: rate between 150 and 250/min, may not be visible, may be merged into preceding T waves; if visible, different morphology from sinus P waves.
- *Relationship between P waves and QRS complexes*: difficult to ascertain relationship; PR interval often cannot be determined because P waves are not clearly distinguishable; if there is AV block, P waves may not be conducted to the ventricles (usually 2:1 AV block, i.e. every other P wave is blocked).

### Effects on the patient

Atrial tachycardia may be associated with palpitations or haemo-dynamic compromise due to the loss of effective atrial contractions and a rapid ventricular rate. In severe cases, the patient may become confused due to cerebral hypoxaemia (Docherty, 2002).

### Treatment

The patient should be assessed following the ABCDE approach, support ABCs, administer oxygen and insert an intravenous cannula; monitor blood pressure, the ECG and oxygen saturations; ideally record a 12 lead ECG, if unable to do so print off an ECG rhythm strip; identify and treat underlying causes, e.g. correct electrolyte abnormalities (Resuscitation Council UK, 2006). If the patient is stable, use vagal manoeuvres and adenosine (see pages 226–27). If the patient is taking digoxin, toxicity should be suspected and the digoxin should be omitted (Bennett, 2006). If the patient is unstable, synchronised electrical cardioversion is recommended (Resuscitation Council UK, 2006).

### Interpretation of Figure 5.4

- *Electrical activity*: present.
- *QRS rate*: 180/min.
- *QRS rhythm*: regular.
- *QRS width*: normal width and constant morphology.
- *P waves*: present on the preceding T waves.

- *Relationship between P waves and QRS complexes*: each P wave is followed by a QRS complex and each QRS complex is preceded by a P wave; PR interval constant.

The ECG in Figure 5.4 displays atrial tachycardia. The patient was admitted to the coronary ward with palpitations. There were no adverse signs present and the patient was stable (see page 78). Carotid sinus massage applied by the doctor was ineffective. Adenosine 6 mg was then administered IV, but without success. Three further doses of 12 mg each were also unsuccessful. As there were no adverse signs present (i.e. patient did not require cardioversion at that stage), amiodarone 300 mg was administered IV over one hour. This was successful at terminating the arrhythmia. The patient's haemodynamic status was monitored throughout in order to promptly detect the presence of adverse signs that would indicate that the patient was becoming unstable.

## ATRIAL FLUTTER
Atrial flutter is less common than atrial fibrillation and is nearly always associated with significant cardiac disease, e.g. mitral valve disease (Nolan *et al.*, 1998). It complicates 2–5% of acute myocardial infarctions (Marriott & Meyerburg, 1986). It usually arises in the right atrium and is often associated with diseases of the right side of the heart, e.g. COPD, massive pulmonary embolism and chronic congestive heart failure (Resuscitation Council UK, 2006).

It is characterised by a zigzagging baseline which produces the typical sawtooth flutter (F) waves, often most evident in the inferior leads and in lead V1 (Goodacre & Irons, 2008). If this characteristic pattern is not initially obvious, it can be frequently visualised by applying carotid sinus massage to increase AV block (Thompson, 1997).

Atrial flutter is often initiated by an atrial premature beat and may degenerate into atrial fibrillation (Bennett, 2006). In the majority of cases the atrial rate is 300/min and only alternate F waves are conducted to the ventricles (2:1 AV block) (Camm & Katritsis, 1996; Goodacre & Irons, 2008); the presence of a regular tachycardia rate 150/min suggests the possible diagnosis of atrial flutter (Goodacre & Irons, 2008).

## Identifying features on the ECG

- *Electrical activity*: present.
- *QRS rate*: dependent on the degree of AV block; usually 150/ min.
- *QRS rhythm*: regular or irregular (dependent on AV block).
- *QRS width*: normal width and constant morphology.
- *P waves*: sawtooth flutter waves present, usually 300/min; best seen in inferior leads.
- *Relationship between P waves and QRS complexes*: usually a degree of AV block is present, e.g. 2:1, 3:1 and 4:1 AV block; AV block may be variable.

### Effects on the patient

Patients with atrial flutter usually present with rapid palpitations (Camm & Katritsis, 1996). Sometimes atrial flutter is associated with haemodynamic compromise owing to the loss of effective atrial contractions and a rapid ventricular rate (Nolan *et al.*, 1998).

### Treatment

Atrial flutter usually responds to carotid sinus massage, most commonly with a decrease in ventricular rate (rarely atrial fibrillation or sinus rhythm) (Camm & Katritsis, 1996).

Although class 1 anti-arrhythmic drugs, e.g. sotolol, flecainide and disopyramide, may terminate atrial flutter, if unsuccessful they may actually lead to 1:1 conduction and higher ventricular rates (Bennett, 2006). Amiodarone is often effective (Nolan *et al.*, 1998) and synchronised cardioversion is very effective (De Silva *et al.*, 1980). Overdrive atrial pacing can restore sinus rhythm in 70% of patients (Nolan *et al.*, 1998). Catheter ablation has also been shown to be effective (Saoudi *et al.*, 1990). Any electrolyte imbalances should be corrected.

### Interpretation of Figure 5.5

- *Electrical activity*: present.
- *QRS rate*: 110/min.
- *QRS rhythm*: irregular owing to varying AV block.
- *QRS width*: normal width and constant morphology.
- *P waves*: flutter waves present 300/min.

- *Relationship between P waves and QRS complexes*: not every flutter wave is followed by a QRS complex but every QRS complex is preceded by a flutter wave; varying degrees of AV block present.

The ECG in Figure 5.5 displays atrial flutter with varying degrees of AV block. This patient was haemodynamically stable and there were no adverse signs. Unfortunately, amiodarone was ineffective at terminating the arrhythmia. However, following synchronised cardioversion at 100 J, sinus rhythm was restored.

### Interpretation of Figure 5.6

- *Electrical activity*: present.
- *QRS rate*: 90/min.
- *QRS rhythm*: regular.
- *QRS width*: normal width and constant morphology.
- *P waves*: flutter waves present, rate 270/min.
- *Relationship between P waves and QRS complexes*: not every flutter wave is followed by a QRS complex but every QRS complex is preceded by a flutter wave; 3:1 AV block present.

The ECG in Figure 5.6 displays atrial flutter with 3:1 AV block. This patient was not haemodynamically compromised. There were no adverse signs and BP was stable. Amiodarone 300 mg was administered IV over one hour which was effective at terminating the arrhythmia.

### Interpretation of Figure 5.7

- *Electrical activity*: present.
- *QRS rate*: 150/min.
- *QRS rhythm*: regular.
- *QRS width*: normal width and constant morphology.
- *P waves*: flutter waves present, rate 300/min.
- *Relationship between P waves and QRS complexes*: not every flutter wave is followed by a QRS complex but every QRS complex is preceded by a flutter wave; 2:1 AV block present.

The ECG in Figure 5.7 displays atrial flutter with 2:1 AV block. The constant ventricular rate of 150 per minute is suggestive of the diagnosis. Careful examination of the 12 lead ECG recorded in this patient (see ECG 22, page 271) confirms the diagnosis: note

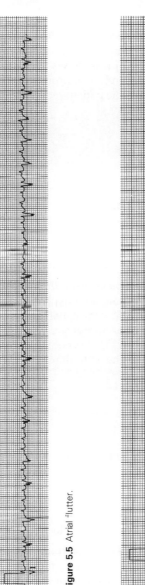

**Figure 5.5** Atrial flutter.

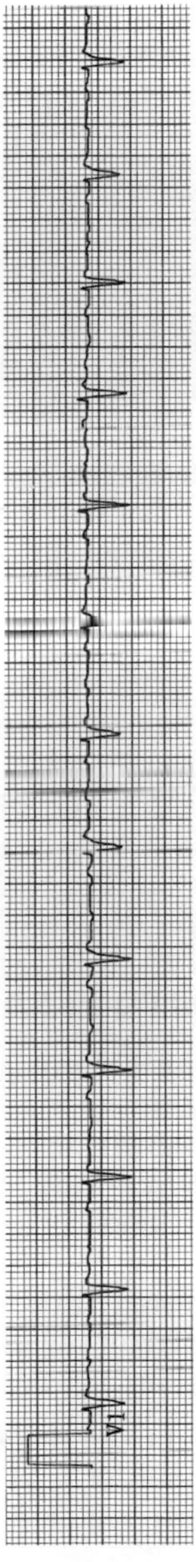

**Figure 5.6** Atrial flutter.

the flutter waves in V1 (there are also widespread ischaemic changes (ST segment depression). This ECG was recorded in a 54-year-old male. He complained of chest tightness, was drowsy, clammy, pale and his blood pressure was unrecordable (severe adverse signs). He was severely compromised. The cardiology registrar was fast bleeped as the patient required urgent electrical cardioversion.

### Interpretation of Figure 5.8

- *Electrical activity*: present.
- *QRS rate*: 100/min.
- *QRS rhythm*: irregular.
- *QRS width*: normal width and constant morphology.
- *P waves*: flutter waves present, rate 300/min.
- *Relationship between P waves and QRS complexes*: not every flutter wave is followed by a QRS complex but every QRS complex is preceded by a flutter wave; varying degrees of AV block present.

The ECG in Figure 5.8 displays atrial flutter with variable AV block. This patient had dilated cardiomyopathy and was acutely short of breath. Although the ventricular rate was not unduly fast, amiodarone 300mg was administered IV over one hour, followed by 900mg IV over 24 hours. This treatment regime was effective at terminating the arrhythmia.

### Interpretation of Figure 5.9

- *Electrical activity*: present.
- *QRS rate*: 300/min.
- *QRS rhythm*: regular.
- *QRS width*: 160ms wide, constant morphology. Right bundle branch block pattern.
- *P waves*: flutter waves present, rate 300/min.
- *Relationship between P waves and QRS complexes*: not every flutter wave is followed by a QRS complex but every QRS complex is preceded by a flutter wave; 1:1 AV block present.

The ECG in Figure 5.9 displays atrial flutter with 1:1 AV block. Careful examination of lead V1 reveals the flutter waves. This patient would have required urgent review by a cardiologist.

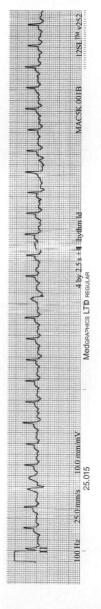

**Figure 5.7** Atrial flutter.

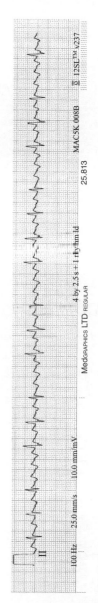

**Figure 5.8** Atrial flutter.

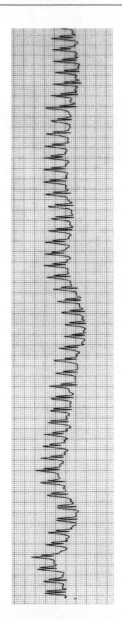

**Figure 5.9** Atrial flutter 1 : 1 conduction.

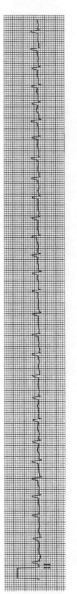

**Figure 5.10** Atrial fibrillation.

## ATRIAL FIBRILLATION

Atrial fibrillation is characterised by rapid re-entrant impulses that result in incomplete contractions and ineffective emptying of the atria (Camm & Katritsis, 1996; Hardin & Steele, 2008). It is usually triggered by an atrial ectopic (Zipes, 1992), though it may result from a degeneration of other supraventricular tachycardias, particularly atrial tachyacrdia and flutter (Goodacre & Irons, 2008). It may be paroxysmal, persistent or permanent (Goodacre & Irons, 2008).

The prevalence of atrial fibrillation increases with age (Lake & Thompson, 1991). It is particularly common amongst older adults (Hardin & Steele, 2008); approximately 5% of individuals older than age 69 and 8% of those older than age 80 will experience it (Rosenthal, 2007).

Causes of atrial fibrillation include valvular heart disease, dilated cardiomyopathy, aortic stenosis, hypertension, ischaemic heart disease, pericarditis, thyrotoxicosis, pulmonary disease, cardiac surgery, alcohol excess and alcohol withdrawal (Hardin & Steele, 2008).

As the atria are not contracting effectively, they do not completely empty of blood; consequently, blood can pool, forming a thrombus (blood clot) which could potentially result in an embolus and a stroke (Hardin & Steele, 2008). It is estimated that 15–25% of all strokes are associated with atrial fibrillation (Rosenthal, 2007).

Classification of atrial fibrillation into three major categories has been proposed by the American College of Cardiology, the American Heart Association and the European Society of Cardiology:

- *First detected atrial fibrillation*: newly diagnosed, the cause will need to be identified.
- *Recurrent atrial fibrillation*: patients who have experienced two or more episodes of atrial fibrillation; categorised as either paroxysmal (ending < 7 days) or chronic (lasting > 7 days). The patient's history is important to determine the appropriate category (Lévy, 2000)
- *Lone atrial fibrillation*: a cardiopulmonary cause can not be identified

(Source: Fuster *et al.*, 2006)

The atria discharge at a rate of 350–600/min (Bennett, 2006). These impulses bombard the AV junction and are intermittently conducted to the ventricles. This results in the characteristic totally irregular QRS rhythm. Sometimes it may be difficult to distinguish atrial fibrillation with a fast ventricular response from other tachycardias. However, the RR interval will be irregular and the overall ventricular rate often fluctuates (Goodacre & Irons, 2008). The ventricular rate will depend on the degree of AV conduction; with normal conduction the rate will be 100–180/min. Slower ventricular rates suggest a higher degree of AV block or the patient may be taking medication that slows conduction in the AV node, e.g. digoxin (Goodacre & Irons, 2008).

### Identifying features on the ECG

- *Electrical activity*: present.
- *QRS rate*: may be slow, normal or rapid.
- *QRS rhythm*: totally irregular (regular if third degree AV block present).
- *QRS width*: usually normal width and constant morphology.
- *P waves*: not present; irregular baseline owing to fibrillation waves.
- *Relationship between P waves and QRS complexes*: not applicable (no P waves present).

### Effects on the patient

The loss of 'atrial kick' (atrial contraction) results in a decrease in cardiac output by as much as 20–30% (Stewart, 2002); this, together with a rapid ventricular response, can lead to a fall in cardiac output of up to 50% (Nolan *et al.*, 1998). Heart failure may occur, particularly if the patient has coexistent valvular heart disease or impaired left ventricular function (Nolan *et al.*, 1998). A significant apical-peripheral pulse deficit may exist when the ventricular rate is rapid (Jevon, 2000).

However, not all patients with atrial fibrillation will exhibit symptoms. Those who do, commonly describe feelings of a rapid or irregular heartbeat, or palpitations or fluttering in the chest (Hardin & Steele, 2008), weakness, shortness of breath, chest pain, feeling faint and syncope (McCabe & Geoffroy, 2002).

If atrial fibrillation persists for more than 48 hours, there is stasis of blood in the fibrillating atria, which can lead to clot formation (Nolan *et al.*, 1998). This results in an increased risk of systemic thromboembolism (Wolf *et al.*, 1991). In long-term atrial fibrillation, warfarin is often administered prophylactically against embolisation (BNF 52, 2006).

## Treatment
Treatment should take into account the clinical setting in which atrial fibrillation occurs; any remediable factors should be addressed if possible. The treatment is aimed at:

- Slowing down the ventricular response.
- Converting it to sinus rhythm (if possible).
- Reducing the frequency and haemodynamic effects of subsequent atrial fibrillation or preventing further episodes.
- Correcting any electrolyte imbalances

Possible drug therapy includes digoxin and amiodarone. Synchronised electrical cardioversion is used when the patient becomes unstable or drug therapy has failed to convert the patient to a normal sinus rhythm. The goals of treatment are to control the heart rate and rhythm and to prevent an embolism occurring (de Denus *et al.*, 2005; Singer *et al.*, 2004; St-Louis & Robichaud-Ekstrand, 2003). Most patients will receive anti-thrombotic therapy, e.g. heparin, low-molecular weight heparin and warfarin.

## Interpretation of Figure 5.10
- *Electrical activity*: present.
- *QRS rate*: 160/min.
- *QRS rhythm*: irregular.
- *QRS width*: normal width and constant morphology.
- *P waves*: none present.
- *Relationship between P waves and QRS complexes*: not applicable (P waves not present).

The ECG in Figure 5.10 displays atrial fibrillation with a rapid ventricular response. This patient developed atrial fibrillation as a complication of myocardial infarction. On assessment, the patient was pale, clammy, dyspnoeic and agitated; BP was 80/55.

These adverse signs of poor cardiac output indicated that the patient was haemodynamically compromised. Urgent electrical cardioversion was required.

### Interpretation of Figure 5.11

- *Electrical activity*: present.
- *QRS rate*: 190/min.
- *QRS rhythm*: irregular.
- *QRS width*: normal width and constant morphology.
- *P waves*: none present.
- *Relationship between P waves and QRS complexes*: not applicable (P waves not present).

The ECG in Figure 5.11 displays atrial fibrillation with a rapid ventricular response. This patient presented to accident and emergency with a four-hour history of palpitations. On assessment, the patient was pale, clammy, dyspnoeic and drowsy; BP was 70/45. Urgent electrical cardioversion was required.

### Interpretation of Figure 5.12

- *Electrical activity*: present.
- *QRS rate*: 190/min.
- *QRS rhythm*: irregular.
- *QRS width*: normal width and constant morphology.
- *P waves*: none present.
- *Relationship between P waves and QRS complexes*: not applicable (P waves not present).

The ECG in Figure 5.12 displays atrial fibrillation with a rapid ventricular response. This patient was complaining of palpitations, but although the ventricular rate was rapid, he was surprisingly not haemodynamically compromised. The patient was started on IV amiodarone and the cardiology registrar was asked to review the patient.

### Interpretation of Figure 5.13

- *Electrical activity*: present.
- *QRS rate*: 140/min.
- *QRS rhythm*: irregular.

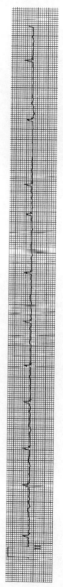

**Figure 5.11** Atrial fibrillation.

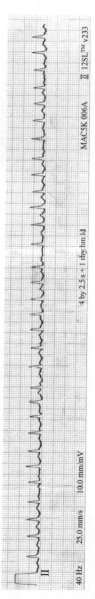

**Figure 5.12** Atrial fibrillation.

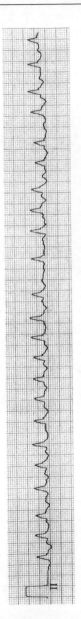

**Figure 5.13** Atrial fibrillation with aberrant conduction.

- *QRS width*: 140 ms (aberrant conduction), constant morphology.
- *P waves*: none present.
- *Relationship between P waves and QRS complexes*: not applicable (P waves not present).

The ECG in Figure 5.13 displays atrial fibrillation with a rapid ventricular response. There is aberrant conduction. The patient was complaining of palpitations, but did not have any adverse signs. He was started on IV amiodarone and the cardiology registrar was asked to review the patient.

## CHAPTER SUMMARY
Cardiac arrhythmias originating in the atria are generally caused by either ischaemic damage to, or over distension of, the atrial walls. If present, P waves are of different morphology from sinus P waves. As the ventricles are activated via the normal conduction pathways, the QRS complex is usually narrow and of a normal morphology. The recognition of APBs, atrial tachycardia, atrial flutter and atrial fibrillation has been described in this chapter.

## REFERENCES
BNF 52 (2006) *British National Formulary*. British Medical Association & Royal Pharmaceutical Society of Great Britain, London.

Bennett DH (2006) *Cardiac Arrhythmias*, 6th edn. Butterworth Heinemann, Oxford.

Camm A, Katritsis D (1996) The diagnosis of tachyarrhythmias. In: Julian D, Camm, AJ, Fox KM, *et al.* (eds) *Diseases of the Heart*, 2nd edn. W.B. Saunders, London.

de Denus S, Sanoski C, Carlsson J, Opolski G, Spinler S (2005) Rate vs rhythm control in patients with atrial fibrillation: a meta-analysis. *Archives of Internal Medicine*, **165**, 258–262.

De Silva R, Graboys T, Podrid P, Lown B (1980) Cardioversion and defibrillation. *American Heart Journal*, **100**, 881–895.

Docherty B (2002) Cardiorespiratory physical assessment for the acutely ill: part 1. *British Journal of Nursing*, **11** (11), 750–758.

Docherty B (2003) 12 lead ECG interpretation and chest pain management. *British Journal of Nursing*, **12** (21), 1248–1255.

Fuster V, Rydén LE, Cannom DS, *et al.* (2006) ACC/AHA/ESC 2006 guidelines for the management of patients with atrial fibrillation: a report of the American College of Cardiology/American Heart Association Task Force on Practice Guidelines and the European Society of Cardiology Committee for Practice Guidelines (Writing Committee to Revise the 2001 Guidelines for the Management of Patients With Atrial Fibrillation): developed in collaboration with the European Heart Rhythm Association and the Heart Rhythm Society. *Circulation*, **114**, e257–e354.

Goodacre S, Irons R (2008) Atrial arrhythmias. In: Morris F, Brady W, Camm J (eds) *ABC of Clinical Electrocardiography*, 2nd edn. Blackwell Publishing, Oxford.

Hardin S, Steele J (2008) Atrial fibrillation among the elderly. *Journal of Gerontological Nursing*, **34** (7), 26–33.

Jevon P (2000) Cardiac monitoring. *Nursing Times*, **96** (23), 43–44.

Harrigan R, Jones K (2008) Conditions affecting the right side of the heart. In: Morris F, Brady W, Camm J (eds) *ABC of Clinical Electrocardiography*, 2nd edn. Blackwell Publishing, Oxford.

Houghton A, Gray D (2003) *Making Sense of the ECG: a Hands on Guide*, 2nd edn. Hodder Arnold, London.

Julian D, Cowan J (1993) *Cardiology*, 6th edn. Baillière, London.

Lake F, Thompson P (1991) Prevention of embolic complications in non-valvular atrial fibrillation in the elderly. *Drugs and Aging*, **1** (6), 458–466.

Lévy S (2000) Classification system of atrial fibrillation. *Current Opinion in Cardiology*, **15**, 54–57.

McCabe P, Geoffroy S (2002) Atrial fibrillation: the newest frontier in arrhythmia management. *Progress in Cardiovascular Nursing*, **17**, 110–123.

Marriott HJL (1988) *Practical Electrocardiography*, 8th edn. Williams & Wilkins, London.

Marriott H, Meyerburg R (1986) Recognition of arrhythmias and conduction abnormalities. In Hurst J (ed.) *The Heart, Arteries and Veins*. McGraw-Hill, New York.

Meltzer LE, Pinneo R, Kitchell JR (1983) *Intensive Coronary Care: a Manual for Nurses*, 4th edn. Prentice Hall, London.

Nolan J, Greenwood J, Mackintosh A (1998) *Cardiac Emergencies: a Pocket Guide*. Butterworth Heinemann, Oxford.

Resuscitation Council UK (2006) *Advanced Life Support*, 5th edn. Resuscitation Council UK, London.

Rosenthal L (2007) *Atrial Fibrillation*: from the eMedicine web site: http://www.emedicine.com (accessed 14 April 2007)

Saoudi N, Attalah G, Kirkorian G, Touboul P (1990) Catheter ablation of the atrial myocardium in human type 1 atrial flutter. *Circulation*, **81**, 762–771.

Singer D, Albers G, Dalen J, *et al.* (2004) Antithrombotic therapy in atrial Fibrillation. *Chest*, **126** (3 Suppl.), 429S–456S.

Soanes C, Stevenson A (2006) *Oxford Dictionary of English*. Oxford University Press, Oxford.

St-Louis L, Robichaud-Ekstrand S (2003) Knowledge level and coping strategies according to coagulation levels in older persons with atrial fibrillation. *Nursing & Health Sciences*, **5**, 67–75.

Stewart S (2002) Atrial fibrillation in the twenty-first century: the new cardiac 'Cinderella' and new horizons for cardiovascular nursing? *European Journal of Cardiovascular Nursing*, **1**, 115–121.

Thompson P (1997) *Coronary Care Manual*. Churchill Livingstone, London.

Wolf P, Abbot R, Kannel W (1991) Atrial fibrillation as an independent risk factor for stroke: the Framlington Study. *Stroke*, **22**, 983–988.

Zipes D (1992) Genesis of cardiac arrhythmias: electrophysiological considerations. In: Braunwald E (ed.) *Heart Disease: a Textbook of Cardiovascular Medicine*, 4th edn. W.B. Saunders, Philadelphia.

# 6 | Cardiac Arrhythmias Originating in the AV Junction

## INTRODUCTION
Cardiac arrhythmias originating in the AV junction can be caused by suppression of the SA node, increased automaticity, re-entry mechanisms or blocking of the impulses in the AV junction itself. The inherent pacing rate of the AV junction is 40–60 beats/min. During junctional arrhythmias the loss of atrial kick can result in a fall in cardiac output of 20–30% (Guyton, 1992).

AV re-entrant tachycardia occurs as a result of an anatomically distinct AV connection (e.g. bundle of Kent in Wolff-Parkinson-White syndrome), which permits the atrial impulse to bypass the AV node and junction and depolarise the ventricles early (ventricular pre-excitation) (Esberger *et al.*, 2008).

The aim of this chapter is to be able to recognise cardiac arrhythmias originating in the AV junction.

## LEARNING OUTCOMES
At the end of the chapter the reader will be able to discuss the characteristic ECG features, list the causes and outline the treatment of:

❑ AV junctional ectopics.
❑ AV junctional escape beats.
❑ AV junctional escape rhythm.
❑ AV junctional tachycardia.

## AV JUNCTIONAL ECTOPICS
AV junctional ectopics are caused by a focus in the AV junction firing earlier in the cardiac cycle than the next timed beat would be expected (Bennett, 2006; Camm & Katritsis, 1996). They are less common than atrial and ventricular ectopics (Bennett, 2006).

They can be a normal finding and can be worsened by cardiac stimulants, e.g. tobacco, caffeine and alcohol (Thompson, 1997).

AV junctional ectopics are characterised by premature QRS complexes, which are of the same morphology as those associated with sinus beats. The impulses are conducted retrogradely to the atria and antegradely to the ventricles. Consequently, the P waves are negative in the inferior leads and positive in aVR. The timing of the P waves in relation to the QRS complexes simply depends on whether the impulses reach the atria or ventricles first (Houghton & Gray, 2003); i.e. the P waves may occur immediately before, during or following the QRS complexes (Camm & Katritsis, 1996).

### Identifying features on the ECG

- *Electrical activity*: present.
- *QRS rate*: determined by the underlying rhythm.
- *QRS rhythm*: slightly irregular owing to junctional premature beats.
- *QRS width*: usually normal width and same morphology as the QRS complexes associated with sinus beats; however, the prematurity of the beat may result in the impulse being conducted to the ventricles with aberration; junctional ectopics occur before the next anticipated sinus beat.
- *P waves*: usually absent; if present they will be of different morphology from those associated with sinus beats, will usually be of opposite polarity to the QRS complexes (upright in V1 or inverted in lead II) and will be located immediately prior to or following the QRS complex.
- *Relationship between P waves and QRS complexes*: if P waves present they occur immediately prior to or following the QRS complexes; if measurable, PR interval is short.

### Effects on the patient

The patient is usually aware of a junctional premature beat, of the subsequent pause often described as a 'missed beat' or of a stronger post-ectopic beat (Camm & Katritsis, 1996). The beats are more evident at night when the patient is in a left lateral position, during or immediately following exercise and while sitting quietly (Camm & Katritsis, 1996). On rare occasions the patient may experience chest pain. Sometimes the patient is asymptomatic.

**Treatment**

Treatment is usually not required (Bennett, 2006). Any electrolyte imbalances should be corrected.

**Interpretation of Figure 6.1**

- *Electrical activity*: present.
- *QRS rate*: 70/min.
- *QRS rhythm*: slightly irregular owing to presence of junctional premature beats.
- *QRS width*: the junctional ectopics are of normal width and the same morphology as the sinus beats; they occur prematurely before the next anticipated sinus beat and are followed by a compensatory pause.
- *P waves*: none associated with the junctional ectopics.
- *Relationship between P waves and QRS complexes*: no P waves associated with junctional ectopics.

The ECG in Figure 6.1 displays sinus rhythm with junctional ectopics. The monitoring lead is lead II and the ST elevation is suggestive of acute myocardial infarction (12 lead ECG was required to help confirm this diagnosis). The absence of P waves, but normal width QRS complexes identical to those associated with the sinus beats, confirms that the ectopic focus is sited in the AV junction. The patient's blood pressure remained stable and there were no adverse affects. No treatment was required.

## AV JUNCTIONAL ESCAPE BEATS

If the SA node fails to discharge, escape beats will normally arise from a subsidiary pacemaker, usually the AV junction. Junctional escape beats are not a primary diagnosis; they are symptomatic of an underlying primary disturbance to which they are secondary (Marriott, 1988 and Jevon, 2002).

Following a long pause in the cardiac cycle, junctional escape beats 'rescue' the heart from cardiac standstill. To quote Professor Marriott (1988), an escape beat 'is a rescuing beat – a friend in need – and as such, of course, should never be treated'.

The SA node usually recovers and resumes its role as pacemaker immediately following a junctional escape beat. Sometimes a series of junctional escape beats occur; six or more are commonly termed junctional escape rhythm or idiojunctional rhythm.

Junctional escape beats are characterised by late QRS complexes, which are similar in appearance to those occurring in sinus rhythm. They occur later than the expected sinus beat. They are not usually associated with retrograde conduction (Marriott, 1988). It is important to distinguish between premature beats and escape beats because the latter suggests impaired pacemaker function (Bennett, 2006).

### Identifying features on the ECG

- *Electrical activity*: present.
- *QRS rate*: determined by underlying rhythm.
- *QRS rhythm*: irregular owing to pauses.
- *QRS width*: usually normal width and same morphology as the QRS complexes associated with sinus beats; junctional escape beats occur later than the next anticipated sinus beat.
- *P waves*: usually absent; if present are of different morphology from those associated with sinus beats, are of opposite polarity to the QRS complexes (upright in V1 or inverted in lead II) and occur immediately prior to or following the QRS complex.
- *Relationship between P waves and QRS complexes*: if P waves present they occur immediately prior to or following the QRS complexes; if measurable, PR interval is short.

### Effects on the patient

Depending on the length of the preceding pause, the patient may complain of lightheadedness or dizziness.

### Treatment

Junctional escape beats themselves do not require treatment. They should not be suppressed by drugs (Bennett, 2006). However, atropine is sometimes administered to speed up the underlying rhythm. Investigations may be required to establish the cause of SA node failure. Medications such as beta blockers may need to be withdrawn or have their dose reduced. Any electrolyte imbalances should be corrected.

### Interpretation of Figure 6.2

- *Electrical activity*: present.
- *QRS rate*: 50/min.

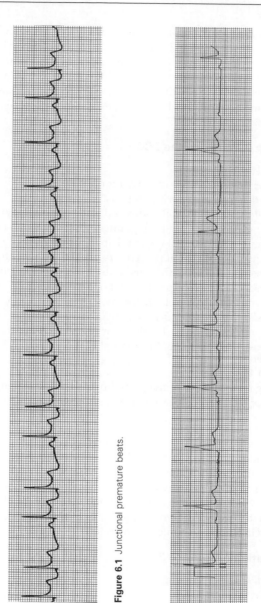

**Figure 6.1** Junctional premature beats.

**Figure 6.2** Junctional escape beats.

- *QRS rhythm*: irregular owing to pauses.
- *QRS width*: the QRS complexes in the underlying rate are wide (0.12 s/3 small squares); the junctional escape beat is of normal width and expected morphology for lead II.
- *P waves*: none associated with junctional escape beat; otherwise present and constant morphology.
- *Relationship between P waves and QRS complex*: AV dissociation.

The ECG in Figure 6.2 displays third degree AV block with a ventricular escape rhythm. The ventricular rhythm is unusually rapid (50/min). However, an almost 2 s pause results in a junctional escape beat. As a rule, the inherent junctional rhythm is faster than its ventricular counterpart. On this occasion, however, it is slower, perhaps because the patient had an acute inferior myocardial infarction (increased vagal tone affecting the AV junction). No treatment was required as sinus rhythm quickly ensued.

## AV JUNCTIONAL ESCAPE RHYTHM

Junctional escape rhythm is said to be present when there are six or more consecutive junctional escape beats. It can occur if the SA node fails to initiate impulses. It is not a primary diagnosis, rather a symptom of an underlying primary disturbance to which it is secondary. It is often initiated with a junctional escape beat. The inherent rate of the AV junction is 40–60 beats/min (Channer & Morris, 2008). Junctional escape rhythm begins later than the next anticipated sinus beat and the rate will be slower than the normal sinus rate.

### Identifying features on the ECG

- *Electrical activity*: present.
- *QRS rate*: usually 40–60/min.
- *QRS rhythm*: usually regular.
- *QRS width*: usually normal width and same configuration as the QRS complexes associated with sinus beats.
- *P waves*: usually absent; if present, are of different morphology from those associated with sinus beats, are of opposite polarity to the QRS complexes (upright in V1 or inverted in lead II) and occur immediately prior to or following the QRS complex.

- *Relationship between P waves and QRS complexes*: if P waves present they occur immediately prior to or following the QRS complexes; if measurable, PR interval is short.

### Effects on the patient

The patient may be haemodynamically compromised, particularly if the rhythm is sustained. The loss of 'atrial kick' will contribute to the fall in cardiac output.

### Treatment

Junctional escape rhythm itself does not require treatment. It should not be suppressed by drugs (Bennett, 2006). Treatment is aimed at stimulating a higher pacemaker. Sometimes atropine is administered to speed up the underlying rhythm. Pacing may be required. The cause of SA node failure should be sought, e.g. medications, myocardial ischaemia/infarction. Any electrolyte imbalances should be corrected.

### Interpretation of Figure 6.3

- *Electrical activity*: present.
- *QRS rate*: 35/min.
- *QRS rhythm*: regular.
- *QRS width*: normal width and morphology constant.
- *P waves*: on this lead unable to identify any P waves; a 12 lead ECG would probably highlight them situated on the T waves.
- *Relationship between P waves and QRS complexes*: not applicable.

The ECG in Figure 6.3 displays junctional escape rhythm. This patient was taking beta blockers which may explain why the junctional rhythm is unusually slow. Although the QRS rate was slow, there were no other adverse signs. The BP was 110/70. The beta blocker was temporarily omitted and sinus rhythm rapidly ensued. No further treatment was required.

### Interpretation of Figure 6.4

- *Electrical activity*: present.
- *QRS rate*: 50/min.
- *QRS rhythm*: regular.
- *QRS width*: normal width and constant morphology.

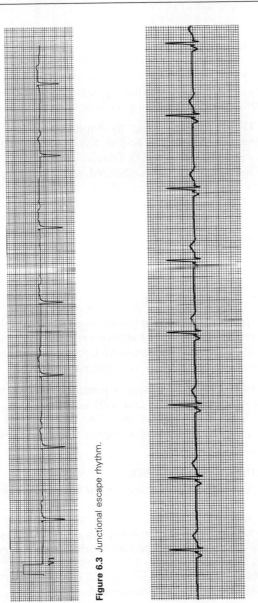

**Figure 6.3** Junctional escape rhythm.

**Figure 6.4** Junctional escape rhythm.

- *P waves*: present but inverted.
- *Relationship between P waves and QRS complexes*: each P wave is followed by a QRS complex and each QRS complex is preceded by a P wave; abnormally short PR interval together with inverted (instead of expected upright) P waves implying retrograde conduction to the atria from the AV junction.

The ECG in Figure 6.4 (lead II) displays junctional escape rhythm. Inverted P waves in lead II, together with a short PR interval, are characteristic ECG features of junctional escape rhythm. This patient had been admitted with a suspected myocardial infarction. There were no adverse signs and the BP was 115/80. No treatment was required. Continuous cardiac monitoring was started.

### Interpretation of Figure 6.5

- *Electrical activity*: present.
- *QRS rate*: 60/min.
- *QRS rhythm*: regular.
- *QRS width*: normal width and constant morphology.
- *P waves*: present but inverted (note the upright P wave in aVR)
- *Relationship between P waves and QRS complexes*: each P wave is followed by a QRS complex and each QRS complex is preceded by a P wave; the PR interval is within normal limits.

The ECG in Figure 6.5 displays junctional escape rhythm. Inverted P waves in lead II and aVR are characteristic ECG features of junctional escape rhythm. The PR interval is within normal limits. This patient was asymptomatic and no treatment was required.

### AV JUNCTIONAL TACHYCARDIA

AV junctional tachycardia is characterised by a sudden onset, an abrupt end, a regular rhythm and a rate of 180–200 beats/min (Camm & Katritsis, 1996 and Jevon & Ewens, 2007). The QRS complexes are of the same morphology as those associated with sinus beats (unless there is aberrant conduction or an existing conduction defect).

Tachycardia related ST depression is frequently evident, which may persist following the termination of the arrhythmia, but is not significant (Nolan *et al.*, 1998). Abnormal (retrograde) P waves may be present. However, in the majority of cases, atrial and ventricular depolarisation occurs simultaneously, with the resultant P waves either superimposed on, or hidden in, the QRS complexes.

AV junctional tachycardia is normally caused by a re-entry mechanism, triggered activity or enhanced automaticity (Esberger *et al.*, 2008).

## Identifying features on the ECG

- *Electrical activity*: present.
- *QRS rate*: usually 180–200/min.
- *QRS rhythm*: usually regular.
- *QRS width*: usually normal width and same morphology as the QRS complexes associated with sinus beats (unless aberrant conduction present).
- *P waves*: usually absent; if present they will be of different morphology from those associated with sinus beats and will usually be of opposite polarity to the QRS complexes (upright in V1 or inverted in lead II) and will be located immediately prior to or following the QRS complex.
- *Relationship between P waves and QRS complexes*: if P waves present they occur immediately prior to or following the QRS complexes; if measurable, PR interval is short.

### Effects on the patient
Some patients may be asymptomatic. Most will complain of palpitations. Occasionally the patient may become haemodynamically compromised. This is influenced by the rate, duration of the episode and underlying cardiac disease (Wang *et al.*, 1991).

### Treatment
Vagal manoeuvres may slow or terminate AV junctional tachycardia (Resuscitation Council UK, 2006). Adenosine is often the first drug of choice if there are no contraindications. Atrial pacing and cardioversion are other options if drug therapy fails (Nolan *et al.*, 1998). If the patient is severely compromised and there are adverse signs or if other treatments fail, synchronised electrical cardioversion is usually undertaken. Radio frequency ablation

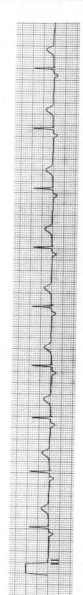

**Figure 6.5** Junctional escape rhythm.

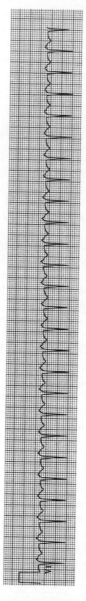

**Figure 6.6** Junctional tachycardia.

may sometimes be required (Nolan *et al.*, 1998). Any electrolyte imbalances should be corrected.

## Interpretation of Figure 6.6

- *Electrical activity*: present.
- *QRS rate*: 150/min.
- *QRS rhythm*: regular.
- *QRS width*: normal width and morphology constant.
- *P waves*: appear to be superimposed on the T waves immediately following the QRS complexes, opposite polarity to the QRS complexes; P waves upright in V1.
- *Relationship between P waves and QRS complexes*: P waves appear to follow QRS complexes (retrograde conduction); PR interval non-existent.

The ECG in Figure 6.6 displays AV junctional tachycardia. Upright P waves in V1 (retrograde conduction from the AV junction) which are of opposite polarity to the QRS complexes (antegrade conduction from the AV junction) help to confirm the diagnosis. This patient was complaining of palpitations but was not haemodynamically compromised. The BP was 135/90 and there were no adverse signs present. The tachycardia did not respond to carotid sinus massage. However, following administration of adenosine, it did revert to sinus rhythm.

## Interpretation of Figure 6.7

- *Electrical activity*: present.
- *QRS rate*: 180/min.
- *QRS rhythm*: regular.
- *QRS width*: normal width and morphology constant.
- *P waves*: none identifiable.
- *Relationship between P waves and QRS complexes*: no identifiable P waves.

The ECG in Fig. 6.7a displays AV junctional tachycardia. The patient was complaining of palpitations but no adverse signs were present. The BP was 108/74. The tachycardia did not respond to carotid sinus massage. However, following adminis-

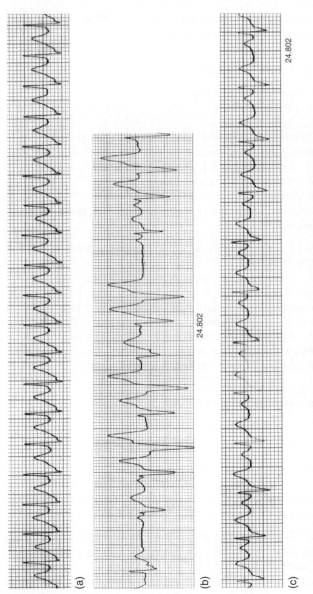

**Figure 6.7** (a) Junctional tachyardia, (b) following administration of adenosine 6 mg IV, (c) and sinus tachycardia.

tration of adenosine 6 mg IV, it did revert to sinus tachycardia with frequent atrial and ventricular ectopics (Figure 6.7b) and then sinus tachycardia rate 110/min (Figure 6.7c).

## Interpretation of Figure 6.8

- *Electrical activity*: present.
- *QRS rate*: 170/min.
- *QRS rhythm*: regular.
- *QRS width*: normal width and morphology constant.
- *P waves*: none identifiable.
- *Relationship between P waves and QRS complexes*: no identifiable P waves.

The ECG in Figure 6.8a displays AV junctional tachycardia. This patient was a 42-year-old lady with a four-hour history of palpitations. When she presented to A & E she was breathless and complaining of chest tightness (note the ST segment depression on the ECG). The tachycardia did not respond to carotid sinus massage. However, following administration of adenosine 6 mg IV and then 12 mg IV it reverted to profound bradycardia (Figure 6.8b) and then sinus rhythm/sinus tachycardia (Figure 6.8c). This reinforces the importance of ensuring the patient is supine on a bed or couch, on an ECG monitor with resuscitation equipment and warning him that he may experience lightheadedness before administering adenosine.

## Interpretation of Figure 6.9

- *Electrical activity*: present.
- *QRS rate*: 150/min.
- *QRS rhythm*: regular.
- *QRS width*: normal width and morphology constant.
- *P waves*: none identifiable.
- *Relationship between P waves and QRS complexes*: no identifiable P waves.

The ECG in Figure 6.9 displays AV junctional tachycardia. This patient was a 65-year-old lady who was complaining of palpitations while receiving chemotherapy. She was also complaining

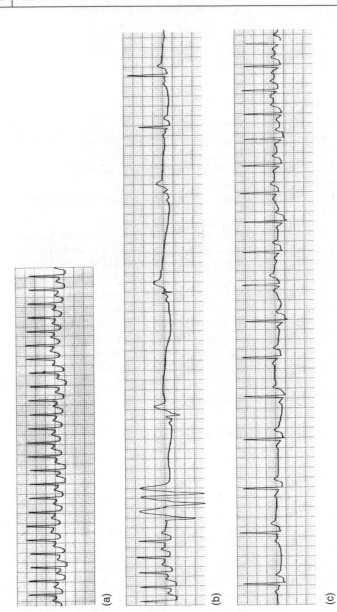

(a)

(b)

(c)

**Figure 6.8** (a) Junctional tachycardia, (b) following administration of adenosine 6 mg and 12 mg IV (c) and sinus tachycardia.

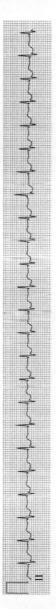

**Figure 6.9** Junctional tachycardia.

of chest tightness: there is ST depression evident. A 12 lead ECG was recorded which showed widespread ischaemic changes. The chemotherapy was temporarily stopped and the cardiologist asked to review the patient.

## CHAPTER SUMMARY

Junctional arrhythmias, which originate in the AV junction, are caused by increased automaticity, suppression of the SA node, re-entry mechanisms or blocking of the impulses in the AV junction itself. Characteristics of junctional arrhythmias include narrow QRS complexes and P waves that are either absent or, if present, immediately precede or follow the QRS complexes. They are usually inverted in leads where they are normally upright and are of opposite polarity to the associated QRS complexes.

## REFERENCES

Bennett DH (2006) *Cardiac Arrhythmias*, 6th edn. Butterworth Heinemann, Oxford.

Camm A, Katritsis D (1996) The diagnosis of tachyarrhythmias. In: Julian D, Camm AJ, Fox KM, *et al.* (eds) *Diseases of the Heart*, 2nd edn. W.B. Saunders, London.

Channer K, Morris F (2008) Myocardial ischaemia. In: Morris F, Brady W, Camm J (eds) *ABC of Clinical Electrocardiography*, 2nd edn. Blackwell Publishing, Oxford.

Esberger D, Jones S, Morris F (2008) Junction tachycardias. In: Morris F, Brady W, Camm J (eds) *ABC of Clinical Electrocardiography*, 2nd edn. Blackwell Publishing, Oxford.

Guyton A (1992) *Human Physiology and Mechanisms of Disease*, 5th edn. W.B. Saunders, Philadelphia.

Houghton A, Gray D (2003) *Making Sense of the ECG: a Hands on Guide*, 2nd edn. Hodder Arnold, London.

Jevon P (2002) *Advanced Cardiac Life Support*, 1st Edn. Butterworth Heinemann, Oxford.

Jevon P, Ewens B (2007) *Monitoring the Critically Ill Patient*, 2nd Edn. Blackwell Publishing, Oxford.

Marriott HJL (1988) *Practical Electrocardiography*, 8th edn. Williams & Wilkins, London.

Nolan J, Greenwood J, Mackintosh A (1998) *Cardiac Emergencies: a Pocket Guide*. Butterworth Heinemann, Oxford.

Resuscitation Council UK (2006) *Advanced Life Support*, 5th Edn. Resuscitation Council (UK), London.

Thompson P (1997) *Coronary Care Manual*. Churchill Livingstone, London.
Wang Y, Scheinman M, Chien W, *et al.* (1991) Patients with supraventricular tachycardia presenting with aborted sudden death: incidence, mechanism and long-term follow-up. *J Am Coll Cardiol*, **18**, 1711.

# 7 | Cardiac Arrhythmias Originating in the Ventricles

## INTRODUCTION

Cardiac arrhythmias originating in the ventricles are commonly caused by an acute myocardial infarction or myocardial ischaemia. Many patients with ischaemic heart disease first present with a ventricular tachyarrhythmia, leading to cardiac arrest and sudden death, without any obvious preceding history of myocardial infarction or angina (Nolan *et al.*, 1998). Other causes of ventricular arrhythmias include cardiac surgery, valvular disease, left ventricular failure, cardiomyopathy and ventricular aneurysm (Bigger, 1991).

The altered pathway of impulse conduction and ventricular depolarisation associated with ventricular arrhythmias results in characteristically wide and bizarre QRS complexes which differ in morphology to QRS complexes associated with the underlying rhythm.

The aim of this chapter is to recognise cardiac arrhythmias originating in the ventricles. Ventricular fibrillation, a cardiac arrhythmia associated with cardiac arrest, is discussed in Chapter 9.

## LEARNING OUTCOMES

At the end of the chapter the reader will be able to discuss the characteristic ECG features, list the causes and outline the treatment for:

❑ Ventricular ectopics.
❑ Ventricular escape beats.
❑ Idioventricular rhythm.
❑ Accelerated idioventricular rhythm.

❑ Ventricular tachycardia.
❑ Torsades de pointes.

## VENTRICULAR ECTOPICS

Ventricular ectopics (VEs), sometimes called ventricular prematture beats (VPBs) or contractions, are caused by an ectopic focus in the ventricles (Docherty, 2003). Causes of ventricular ectopics include ischaemic heart disease, myocardial infarction, electrolyte imbalances and heart failure.

Most ventricular ectopics are wide (0.12 s/3 small squares or more) and bizarre in shape. This is caused by depolarisation across the ventricle walls, which increases the time for contraction to occur, as opposed to the normal His-Purkinje systems. The QRS morphology of the VE differs from that of the QRS complex associated with the underlying rhythm. Generally, an ectopic originating in the left ventricle has a right bundle branch block appearance (positive in V1), and one originating in the right ventricle has a left bundle branch block appearance (negative in V1). The ST segment usually slopes in a direction opposite to the QRS deflection (Camm & Katritsis, 1996). A conducted retrograde P wave may be identifiable in the ST segment/T wave. A full compensatory pause will usually follow – the term 'compensatory pause' is so called because the cycle following the ventricular ectopic compensates for its prematurity and the sinus rhythm then resumes on schedule (Marriott, 1988).

### Ventricular ectopic terminology

- *Uniform or unifocal VEs*: VEs of the same morphology (see Figures 7.1 and 7.2).
- *Multiform*: two or more VEs of distinctly different morphology (the use of the term 'multifocal' is not recommended because impulses from the same focus may be conducted differently (Camm & Katritsis, 1996) (see Figure 7.3).
- *R on T VPB*: a VE which 'lands' on the T wave.
- *Ventricular bigeminy*: a VE after every sinus beat.
- *Ventricular trigeminy*: a VE after every two sinus beats.
- *Couplets*: pairs of VEs (see Figure 7.4).
- *Salvos*: three or more consecutive VEs.

### Identifying features on the ECG

- *Electrical activity*: present.
- *QRS rate*: determined by the underlying rhythm.
- *QRS rhythm*: irregular due to presence of ectopics.
- *QRS width*: the VE will be wide (0.12 s/3 small squares or more), bizarre with changing amplitude, morphology and deflection; morphology differs from that of the QRS complexes associated with the underlying rhythm; ST segment usually slopes in a direction opposite to the QRS deflection; occur before the next anticipated sinus beat and are usually followed by a compensatory pause.
- *P waves*: usually none associated with the VEs (situated on the T wave if present – retrograde conduction).
- *Relationship between P waves and QRS complexes*: usually not possible to determine the relationship between P waves and VEs.

### Effects on the patient

The patient is usually aware of the premature beat itself, of the subsequent pause often described as a missed beat, or of a stronger post-ectopic beat (Camm & Katritsis, 1996). VEs are more noticeable at night when the patient is in a left lateral position, during or immediately following exercise and while sitting quietly (Camm & Katritsis, 1996). On rare occasions the patient may experience chest pain. Sometimes the patient is asymptomatic.

They can be associated with a significant fall in stroke volume and are often not pulse-producing; frequent VEs can therefore have significant haemodynamic effects on the patient.

### Treatment

In the 1980s the administration of anti-arrhythmic drugs to suppress VEs in order to try to 'prevent ventricular fibrillation' was common practice. However, the prophylactic treatment of VEs was found to be ineffective and in fact increase mortality (Mac-Mahon *et al.*, 1988). It is now standard practice to treat ventricular fibrillation if it occurs, rather than attempt to suppress the VEs and prevent it. Treatable causes such as electrolyte imbalances and hypoxia should be corrected (Jowett & Thompson, 1995).

Current recommendations for the management of frequent VEs associated with acute myocardial infarction include adequate pain relief, effective treatment of heart failure and correction of any electrolyte imbalance (Nolan *et al.*, 1998).

### Interpretation of Figure 7.1

- *Electrical activity*: present.
- *QRS rate*: underlying rate is 60/min.
- *QRS rhythm*: irregular owing to presence of VPBs.
- *QRS width*: VEs are wide (0.14s/3.5 small squares) and bizarre; VE morphology differs from that of the QRS complexes associated with the underlying rhythm and ST segment slopes in an opposite direction to the QRS deflection; the ectopics occur before the next anticipated sinus beat.
- *P waves*: inverted P waves can be seen on the ascending limb of the T waves of the ectopics, indicating retrograde conduction from the ventricles to the atria; this possibly explains why there isn't a full compensatory pause following the ectopic.
- *Relationship between P waves and QRS complexes*: unable to determine.

The ECG in Figure 7.1 displays sinus rhythm with uniform or unifocal VPBs. The VPBs have identical morphology, indicating that they have been caused by the same ectopic focus in the ventricles. The patient had complained of palpitations. Only isolated VEs were identified on the ECG and no treatment was required. The BP remained stable and there were no adverse signs. The electrolyte levels were within normal limits.

### Interpretation of Figure 7.2

- *Electrical activity*: present.
- *QRS rate*: underlying rate is 65/min.
- *QRS rhythm*: slightly irregular owing to presence of VE.
- *QRS width*: VE is wide (0.14s/3.5 small squares) and bizarre; VPB morphology differs from that of the QRS complexes associated with the underlying rhythm and ST segment slopes in an opposite direction to the QRS deflection; the VE occurs

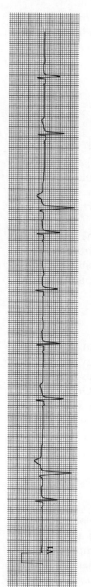

**Figure 7.1** Ventricular premature beats.

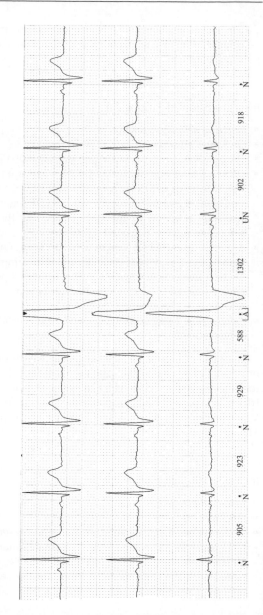

**Figure 7.2** Ventricular ectopic.

before the next anticipated sinus beat and is followed by a full compensatory pause.

- *P waves*: none associated with ventricular ectopics.
- *Relationship between P waves and QRS complexes*: unable to determine.

The ECG in Figure 7.2 displays sinus rhythm with one VE. It was recorded by a 24-hour tape in a patient with a history of palpitations.

### Interpretation of Figure 7.3

- *Electrical activity*: present.
- *QRS rate*: underlying rate is 80/min.
- *QRS rhythm*: slightly irregular owing to presence of VPBs.
- *QRS width*: ventricular ectopics are wide (0.14 s/3.5 small squares) and bizarre; VPB morphology differs from that of the QRS complexes associated with the underlying rhythm and ST segment slopes in an opposite direction to the QRS deflection; ventricular ectopics occur before the next anticipated sinus beat and are followed by a full compensatory pause.
- *P waves*: none associated with ventricular ectopics.
- *Relationship between P waves and QRS complexes*: unable to determine.

The ECG in Figure 7.3 displays sinus rhythm with VEs with varying morphology, suggesting that they have been caused by two ectopic foci in the ventricles. If multi-formed VEs are observed on the ECG, always check serum potassium levels.

### Interpretation of Figure 7.4

- *Electrical activity*: present.
- *QRS rate*: underlying rate is approximately 50/min.
- *QRS rhythm*: irregular due to presence of ventricular ectopics.
- *QRS width*: VEs are wide (0.14 s/3.5 small squares) and bizarre; ventricular ectopic morphology differs from that of the QRS complexes associated with the underlying rhythm and ST segment slopes in an opposite direction to the QRS deflection; ventricular ectopics occur before the next anticipated sinus

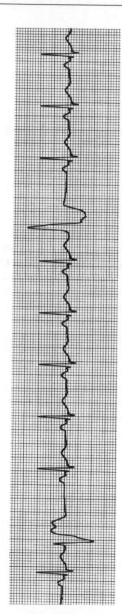

**Figure 7.3** Multi-focal ventricular ectopics.

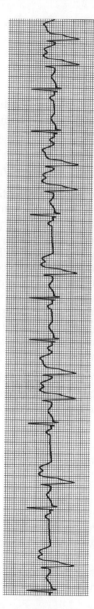

**Figure 7.4** Couplets of ventricular ectopics.

beat and are followed by a full compensatory pause; some ventricular ectopics occur in pairs (couplets).

- *P waves*: are present before the sinus QRS complexes; some are present on VE and are non-conducted.
- *Relationship between P waves and QRS complexes*: normal relationship between the P waves and the sinus QRS complexes; P waves that fall on the T waves of the VEs are non-conducted.

The ECG in Figure 7.4 displays sinus rhythm with unifocal VEs and couplets of VEs. The VEs have identical morphology indicating that they have been caused by the same ectopic focus in the ventricles. A patient presenting with such an ECG may be haemodynamically compromised because of the frequency of the VEs. Oxygen would need to be administered and the patient placed in a semi-recumbent position. Serum potassium level would need to be checked.

## VENTRICULAR ESCAPE BEATS

Ventricular escape beats occur if all potential pacemakers above the ventricles fail to initiate impulses or if these impulses are blocked and fail to reach the ventricles. They are not a primary diagnosis; they are symptomatic of some underlying primary disturbance to which they are secondary (Marriott, 1988). Ventricular escape beats can occur in a variety of settings, including myocardial infarction, digoxin toxicity, overdose of calcium channel blockers or beta blockers and electrolyte disturbances (Purcell, 1993).

In contrast to ventricular ectopics, ventricular escape beats occur later than the next anticipated PQRS complex associated with the underlying rhythm. Following a long pause in the underlying rhythm, ventricular escape beats 'rescue' the heart from cardiac standstill. To quote Marriott (1988), an escape beat 'is a rescuing beat – a friend in need – and as such, of course, should never be treated'.

Ventricular escape beats have similar morphological characteristics to ventricular ectopics; they are wide (0.12 s/3 small squares or more), bizarre in shape and the morphology differs from that of the QRS complexes associated with the underlying rhythm. In general, those originating in the left ventricle have a right bundle branch block appearance (positive in V1), and those originating in the right ventricle have a left bundle branch block appearance (negative in V1). The ST segment usually slopes in a direction opposite to the QRS deflection. They are not usually associated with retrograde conduction (Marriott, 1988).

Normally, the SA node will recover and resume its role as pacemaker immediately following an escape beat. Sometimes a series of escape beats will occur. Six or more ventricular escape beats are commonly termed idioventricular rhythm.

### Identifying features on the ECG

- *Electrical activity*: present.
- *QRS rate*: determined by underlying rhythm.
- *QRS rhythm*: determined by underlying rhythm; presence of ventricular escape beats will result in pauses and an irregular rhythm.
- *QRS width*: usually wide (0.12 s/3 small squares or more) and bizarre, QRS morphology differs from that of the QRS complexes associated with the underlying rhythm; ST segment usually slopes in an opposite direction to the QRS deflection and occurs later than the next anticipated beat, i.e. following a pause in the underlying rhythm.
- *P waves*: usually absent.
- *Relationship between P waves and QRS complexes*: unable to determine.

### Effects on the patient

If there are long pauses the patient may become haemodynamically compromised. The patient may be aware of the pauses.

### Treatment

Ventricular escape beats themselves do not require treatment. They should not be suppressed by drugs (Bennett, 2006). However, atropine is sometimes administered to speed up the underlying rhythm; pacing may be required. The cause of SA node and junctional failure should be established and, if possible, treated. Any electrolyte imbalance should be corrected.

## IDIOVENTRICULAR RHYTHM

An idioventricular rhythm is a series of five or more consecutive ventricular escape beats. It can occur if all potential pacemakers above the ventricles fail to initiate impulses, if the underlying rhythm is slower than the intrinsic ventricular rhythm or if there is third degree AV block. The latter is the most common cause (Purcell, 1993).

Idioventricular rhythm is not a primary diagnosis, rather a symptom of an underlying primary disturbance to which it is secondary. Causes include acute myocardial infarction, reperfusion following thrombolysis, drugs and electrolyte disturbances. The morphology of the QRS complexes is the same as ventricular escape beats. It is often initiated with a ventricular escape beat.

### Identifying features on the ECG

- *Electrical activity*: present
- *QRS rate*: usually 20–40/min.
- *QRS rhythm*: usually regular.
- *QRS width*: usually wide (0.12 s/3 small squares or more) and bizarre; VPD morphology differs from that of the QRS complexes associated with the underlying rhythm; ST segment usually slopes in an opposite direction to the QRS deflection; usually starts after a pause in the underlying rhythm.
- *P waves*: usually absent, though may be present if complete AV block exists.
- *Relationship between P waves and QRS complexes*: AV dissociation if AV block present.

### Effects on the patient

The patient may be haemodynamically compromised, particularly if the rhythm is sustained or slow. The loss of 'atrial kick' will contribute to the fall in cardiac output; however, it is rarely sustained.

### Treatment

Idioventricular rhythm itself does not require treatment. It should not be suppressed by drugs (Bennett, 2006). Treatment is aimed at stimulating a higher pacemaker. Sometimes atropine is administered to speed up the underlying rhythm. Pacing may be required. The cause of SA node and junctional failure should be established and treated if possible. Any electrolyte imbalances should be corrected.

### Interpretation of Figure 7.5

- *Electrical activity*: present.
- *QRS rate*: 30/min.
- *QRS rhythm*: regular.
- *QRS width*: wide (0.16 s/4 small squares) and bizarre; ST segment slopes in an opposite direction to the QRS deflection.
- *P waves*: absent.
- *Relationship between P waves and QRS complexes*: unable to determine.

The ECG in Figure 7.5 displays idioventricular rhythm. The slow rate distinguishes it from accelerated idioventricular rhythm. This patient was admitted with an acute inferior myocardial infarction. His BP was 70/45 and he was pale and clammy. As adverse signs were present, atropine 500 mcg was administered IV, which was successful in speeding up the sinus rate. Idioventricular rhythms associated with inferior myocardial infarction rarely require treatment. However, on this occasion treatment was required because the patient was severely haemodynamically compromised.

### ACCELERATED IDIOVENTRICULAR RYTHM

An accelerated idioventricular rhythm is when an ectopic ventricular focus is discharging at a rate of approximately 100–120/min (Edhouse & Morris, 2008). It is often caused by increased automaticity. AV dissociation is often present until the sinus rate increases sufficiently to regain control of cardiac contraction.

It is frequently associated with myocardial infarction (Hampton, 2000; Lichstein *et al.*, 1976; Nolan *et al.*). It is also often seen during coronary reperfusion following thrombolytic therapy (Miller *et al.*, 1986). It is very similar to idioventricular rhythm except that the rate is faster and AV dissociation is often present.

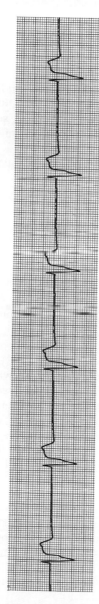

**Figure 7.5** Idioventricular rhythm.

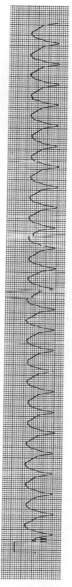

**Figure 7.6** Ventricular tachycardia.

### Identifying features on the ECG

- *Electrical activity*: present.
- *QRS rate*: 100–120/min.
- *QRS rhythm*: usually regular.
- *QRS width*: usually wide (0.12 s/3 small squares or more) and bizarre; VPB morphology differs from that of the QRS complexes associated with the underlying rhythm; ST segment usually slopes in an opposite direction to the QRS deflection.
- *P waves*: often present.
- *Relationship between P waves and QRS complexes*: usually AV dissociation.

### Effects on the patient

An accelerated idioventricular rhythm is normally well tolerated by the patient. It is rarely associated with haemodynamic compromise and rarely degenerates into a life-threatening ventricular tachyarrhythmia (Nolan *et al.*, 1998).

### Treatment

An accelerated idioventricular rhythm is benign and should not be treated (Hampton, 2000).

### VENTRICULAR TACHYCARDIA

Ventricular tachycardia (VT) is commonly associated with ischaemic heart disease, particularly as an early or late consequence of myocardial infarction (Josephson *et al.*, 1978; Wellens *et al.*, 1976). During the acute phase of myocardial infarction, VT commonly deteriorates into ventricular fibrillation and is responsible for a considerable number of sudden cardiac deaths in the community (Camm & Katritsis, 1996). Other causes of VT include cardiomyopathy, electrolyte imbalances and drugs.

VT is diagnosed if there are three or more successive ventricular ectopics at a rate >120 min; it is classed as sustained VT if it lasts for more than 30 seconds and unsustained VT if it lasts for less than 30 seconds (Edhouse & Morris, 2008; Josephson, 1993). The QRS complexes are wide (0.12 s/3 small squares or more) and bizarre. In monomorphic VT the QRS complexes are of constant morphology shape. In polymorphic VT the QRS morphology changes (torsades de pointes, an important variety of this, is discussed in the next section).

In approximately 70% of cases of VT, the atria may continue to depolarise independently of the ventricle, i.e. AV dissociation (Camm & Katritsis, 1996). As this activity is completely independent of ventricular activity, the resultant P waves are dissociated from the QRS complexes and are positive in lead II (Edhouse & Morris, 2008). This independent atrial activity can lead to fusion and capture beats, the presence of which are hallmarks of ventricular tachycardia.

A fusion beat occurs when an impulse from the SA node travelling antegradely meets an impulse from the ventricles travelling retrogradely. The ventricles are therefore depolarised partly by the impulse being conducted through the His-Purkinje system and partly by the impulse arising in the ventricle (Edhouse & Morris, 2008). The QRS complex that results partly resembles a normal complex and partly resembles a VPB complex (Jowett & Thompson, 1995). Fusion beats are uncommon, and although their presence supports a diagnosis of ventricular tachycardia, their absence does not exclude the diagnosis (Edhouse & Morris, 2008).

A capture beat occurs when an impulse from the SA node is conducted to the ventricles, resulting in a P wave followed by a normal QRS complex (Jowett & Thompson, 1995), without otherwise interrupting the arrhythmia (Resuscitation Council UK, 2006). Capture beats are uncommon, and although their presence supports a diagnosis of ventricular tachycardia, their absence does not exclude the diagnosis (Edhouse & Morris, 2008).

Most broad complex tachycardias are ventricular in origin, i.e. ventricular tachycardia. Occasionally a supraventricular tachycardia can be conducted with bundle branch block resulting in a broad complex tachycardia. Twelve lead ECGs should be recorded whenever possible to help confirm diagnosis.

### Identifying features on the ECG

- *Electrical activity*: present.
- *QRS rate*: usually 150–200/min.
- *QRS rhythm*: regular or irregular.

- *QRS width*: wide (0.12 s/3 small squares or more) and bizarre; VPB morphology differs from the QRS complexes associated with the underlying rhythm; ST segment usually slopes in a direction opposite to the QRS deflection.
- *P waves*: may be present.
- *Relationship between P waves and QRS complexes*: if P waves visible, AV dissociation is often present.

### Effects on the patient

Ventricular tachycardia is a serious cardiac arrhythmia. The patient will often be haemodynamically compromised. In some patients cardiac output will be lost. It can degenerate into ventricular fibrillation.

### Treatment

If the patient is pulseless, immediate defibrillation is required. If the patient has a pulse but is haemodynamically compromised, emergency cardioversion is advocated. If the patient is stable, amiodarone is recommended (Resuscitation Council UK, 2006) (see pages 229–37). Any underlying causes, e.g. electrolyte imbalances, should be treated if possible.

### Interpretation of Figure 7.6

- *Electrical activity*: present.
- *QRS rate*: 150/min.
- *QRS rhythm*: regular.
- *QRS width*: wide (0.14 s/3.5 small squares) and bizarre, ST segment slopes in a direction opposite to the QRS deflection.
- *P waves*: some identifiable.
- *Relationship between P waves and QRS complexes*: AV dissociation is present – there is no relationship between the P waves and QRS complexes.

The ECG in Figure 7.6 displays a broad complex tachycardia which is most likely to be ventricular in origin, i.e. ventricular tachycardia. This patient was stable. His BP was 120/70 and he was well perfused. The ventricular rate is only a borderline adverse sign (Resuscitation Council UK, 2006). Amiodarone infusion provided effective treatment. ECG 8 on page 257 depicts a 12 lead ECG recorded in this patient.

## Interpretation of Figure 7.7

- *Electrical activity*: present.
- *QRS rate*: 200/min.
- *QRS rhythm*: regular.
- *QRS width*: wide (0.12s/3 small squares) and bizarre; ST segment slopes in a direction opposite to the QRS deflection.
- *P waves*: not identifiable.
- *Relationship between P waves and QRS complexes*: unable to determine.

The ECG in Figure 7.7 displays a broad complex tachycardia most likely ventricular in origin. A 12 lead ECG would be required to confirm diagnosis. This patient had been admitted to A & E with acute anterior myocardial infarction. He was severely compromised and adverse signs were present. His BP was unrecordable and the patient was semi-conscious. In addition, the rate is very rapid and there is a high risk of degeneration into cardiac arrest. Urgent treatment was required. Synchronised cardioversion was carried out. Successful conversion to sinus rhythm was achieved on the second attempt (200J).

## Interpretation of Figure 7.8

- *Electrical activity*: present.
- *QRS rate*: 210/min.
- *QRS rhythm*: regular/irregular.
- *QRS width*: wide (0.12s/3 small squares) and bizarre; ST segment slopes in a direction opposite to the QRS deflection.
- *P waves*: some are present during the run of ventricular tachycardia.
- *Relationship between P waves and QRS complexes*: AV dissociation.

The ECG in Figure 7.8 displays ventricular tachycardia (self-terminating). It was recorded on a 24-hour ECG tape in a patient with a history of blackouts. Interestingly, following the three-second run of ventricular tachycardia, the ECG shows a period

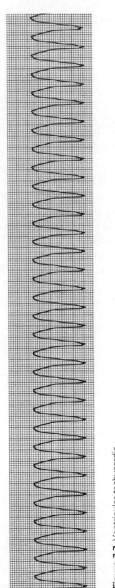

**Figure 7.7** Ventricular tachycardia.

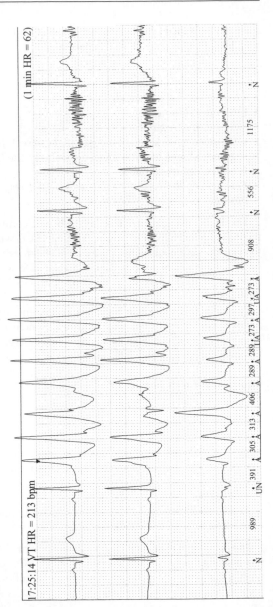

**Figure 7.8** Ventricular tachycardia (self-terminating).

of movement artefact (not present prior to episode), suggesting that the patient was aware of the episode, perhaps even collapsed.

## TORSADES DE POINTES

In 1966, the French physician Francois Dessertenne described a specific electrocardiographic form of polymorphic ventricular tachycardia, which he termed torsades de pointes (Dessertenne, 1966). It refers to an ECG appearance of spiky QRS complexes rotating irregularly around the isoelectric line at a rate of 200–250 beats/min (Dessertenne, 1966).

The word *torsades* refers to an ornamental motif imitating twisted hairs or threads as seen on classical architectural columns, and *pointes* referred to points or peaks (Yap & Camm, 2003). The cardiac axis rotates over a sequence of 5–20 beats, changing from one direction to another and then back again (Edhouse & Morris, 2008).

Torsades de pointes is usually associated with a prolonged QT interval. Causes include anti-arrhythmic drugs, bradycardia due to sick sinus syndrome or AV block, congenital prolongation of the QT interval (e.g. Romano Ward syndrome), hypokalaemia, hypomagnesaemia and tricyclic antidepressant drugs (Bennett, 2006).

It is important to recognise torsades de pointes because the administration of anti-arrhythmic drugs (sometimes administered for monomorphic VT) may actually aggravate it. In addition, correction or removal of the cause may be very effective. Although it is usually non-sustained and repetitive (Bennett, 2006), it can itself cause a cardiac arrest or degenerate into ventricular fibrillation (Resuscitation Council UK, 2006).

### Identifying features on the ECG

- *Electrical activity*: present.
- *QRS rate*: usually 200–250/min.
- *QRS rhythm*: irregular.
- *QRS width*: wide (0.12 s/3 small squares or more) and bizarre, with changing amplitude, morphology and deflection.
- *P waves*: unable to identify.

- *Relationship between P waves and QRS complexes*: AV dissociation may be present.

### Effects on the patient

Torsades de pointes is a very serious cardiac arrhythmia. The patient will often be haemodynamically compromised. In some patients cardiac output will be lost. It can degenerate into ventricular fibrillation.

### Treatment

Effective treatment, i.e. prevention of recurrent episodes, involves removal of any predisposing causes, e.g. drugs, correction of any electrolyte imbalances (Edhouse & Morris, 2008); overdrive pacing may be effective (Resuscitation Council UK, 2006). Measures to speed up the sinus rate may be effective in some situations. If the patient has a cardiac arrest, immediate defibrillation is required.

### Interpretation of Figure 7.9

- *Electrical activity*: present.
- *QRS rate*: 200–250/min.
- *QRS rhythm*: irregular.
- *QRS width*: wide and bizarre, with changing amplitude, morphology and deflection.
- *P waves*: unable to identify.
- *Relationship between P waves and QRS complexes*: unable to determine.

The ECG in Figure 7.9 shows torsades de pointes. It displays the characteristic ECG appearance of spiky QRS complexes rotating irregularly around the isoelectric line. This patient would have required urgent review by a cardiologist.

### CHAPTER SUMMARY

Cardiac arrhythmias originating in the ventricles are characterised by wide, bizarre QRS complexes. Most ventricular tachyarrhythmias are serious. Some can have severe haemodynamic effects on the patient, whereas others can cause a cardiac arrest.

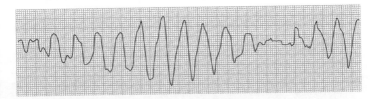

**Figure 7.9** Torsades de pointes. Reprinted from Morris F, *et al.*, *ABC of Clinical Electrocardiography*, 2nd edn, copyright 2008, with permission of Blackwell Publishing.

Their prompt recognition together with appropriate treatment is essential.

REFERENCES

Bennett DH (2006) *Cardiac Arrhythmias*, 4th edn. Butterworth Heinemann, Oxford.

Bigger J (1991) Ventricular dysrhythmias. In: Horowitz, L (ed.) *Current Management of Arrhythmias*. B C Decker, Philadelphia

Camm A, Katritsis D (1996) The diagnosis of tachyarrhythmias. In: Julian D, Camm AJ, Fox KM, *et al.* (eds) *Diseases of the Heart*, 2nd edn. W.B. Saunders, London.

Dessertenne F (1966) La tachycardie ventriculaire a deux foyers opposes variables. *Arch Mal Coeur*, **59**, 263.

Docherty B (2003) 12 lead ECG interpretation and chest pain management. *British Journal of Nursing*, **12** (21), 1248–1255.

Edhouse J, Morris F (2008) Broad complex tachycardia. In: Morris F, Brady W, Camm J (eds) *ABC of Clinical Electrocardiography*, 2nd edn. Blackwell Publishing, Oxford.

Hampton J (2000) *The ECG Made Easy*, 5th edn. Churchill Livingstone, London.

Josephson M (1993) *Clinical Cardiac Electrophysiology*. Lea & Febiger, Philadelphia.

Josephson M, Horowitz L, Farsidi A, Kastor J (1978) Recurrent sustained ventricular tachycardia: 1. Mechanisms. *Circulation*, **57**, 431.

Jowett NI, Thompson DR (1995) *Comprehensive Coronary Care*, 2nd edn. Scutari Press, London.

Lichstein E, Ribas-Meneclier C, Gupta P, Chadda A (1976) Incidence and descriptions of accelerated idioventricular rhythm complicating acute myocardial infarction. *American Journal of Medicine*, **58**, 192–198.

MacMahon S, Collins R, Peto R, *et al.* (1988) Effects of prophylactic lidocaine in suspected myocardial infarction. An overview of results from the randomized controlled trials. *JAMA*, **2601**, 1910–1916.

Marriott HJL (1988) *Practical Electrocardiography*, 8th edn. Williams & Wilkins, London.

Miller F, Kruchoff M, Satler L, *et al.* (1986) Ventricular arrhythmias during reperfusion. *American Heart Journal*, **112**, 928–931.

Nolan J, Greenwood J, Mackintosh A (1998) *Cardiac Emergencies: a Pocket Guide*. Butterworth Heinemann, Oxford.

Purcell J (1993) Cardiac electrical activity. In: Kinney M, Packa D, Dunbar S (eds) *AACN's Clinical Reference for Critical Care Nursing*, 3rd edn. Mosby–Year Book, St Louis.

Resuscitation Council UK (2006) *Advanced Life Support*, 5th edn. Resuscitation Council UK, London.

Wellens H, Durer D, Lie K (1976) Observation on mechanisms of ventricular tachycardia in man. *Circulation*, **54**, 327.

Yap Y, Camm A (2003) Drug induced QT prolongation and torsades de pointes. *Heart*, **89** (11), 1363–1372.

# Cardiac Arrhythmias with Atrioventricular Block

**8**

## INTRODUCTION

Cardiac arrhythmias with AV block can result from a conduction disturbance in the AV node, bundle of His or bundle branches. It is classified as first, second or third degree depending on whether impulse conduction to the ventricles is delayed, intermittently blocked or completely blocked (Bennett, 2006).

Normally, a narrow QRS complex indicates a conduction disturbance in the AV node or bundle of His, whereas a wide QRS complex indicates a conduction disturbance in the bundle branches.

The aim of this chapter is to recognise cardiac arrhythmias with AV block.

## LEARNING OUTCOMES

At the end of the chapter the reader will be able to state the characteristic ECG features, list the causes and outline the treatment of:

❑ First degree AV block.
❑ Second degree AV block Mobitz type 1 (Wenckeback phenomenon).
❑ Second degree AV block Mobitz type 2.
❑ Third degree (complete) AV block.

## FIRST DEGREE AV BLOCK

In first degree AV block, there is a delay, usually in the AV node, in the conduction of atrial impulses to the ventricles (Da Costa *et al.*, 2008). It is characterised by a prolonged, but constant PR interval (>0.20s or 5 small squares), all the impulses are conducted to the ventricles and there are no missed beats (Da Costa *et al.*, 2008). As the impulse is only delayed, not blocked, it could be argued that calling it AV block is misleading.

Although first degree AV block is not in itself important, it may be a sign of coronary heart disease, acute rheumatic carditis, digoxin toxicity or electrolyte imbalance (Hampton, 2000). It can progress to second or third degree AV block. Sometimes it is a normal phenomenon: in young persons it is usually due to increased vagal tone and is benign (Bennett, 2006).

Forty per cent of patients with an acute inferior myocardial infarction and first degree AV block, develop self-terminating well-tolerated episodes of second degree AV block Mobitz type 1 and third degree AV block (Nolan *et al.*, 1998). When associated with an anterior myocardial infarction, it may be the final stage of widespread involvement of the conduction system in a septal infarction (Thompson, 1997).

### Identifying features on the ECG

- *Electrical activity*: present.
- *QRS rate*: usually normal.
- *QRS rhythm*: usually regular.
- *QRS width*: normal width and morphology.
- *P waves*: present and constant morphology.
- *Relationship between P waves and QRS complexes*: each P wave is followed by a QRS complex and each QRS complex is preceded by a P wave; PR interval is prolonged, i.e. >0.20 s/5 small squares.

### Effects on the patient

The patient will be asymptomatic. First degree AV block does not alter the ventricular rate and the abnormality can only be detected on the ECG (Jowett & Thompson, 1995).

### Treatment

It requires no specific treatment, though drugs which can prolong AV conduction, e.g. beta blockers, will probably need to be avoided. However, it is important to monitor the patient closely in case there is progression to a higher degree of AV block.

## Interpretation of Figure 8.1

- *Electrical activity*: present.
- *QRS rate*: 80/min.
- *QRS rhythm*: regular.
- *QRS width*: normal width and morphology.
- *P waves*: present and constant morphology.
- *Relationship between P waves and QRS complexes*: each P wave is followed by a QRS complex and each QRS complex is preceded by a P wave; PR interval is prolonged 0.22s (6 small squares).

The ECG in Figure 8.1 displays first degree AV block. It was only identified following a routine 12 lead ECG. The patient was asymptomatic and no treatment was required.

## Interpretation of Figure 8.2

- *Electrical activity*: present.
- *QRS rate*: 100/min.
- *QRS rhythm*: regular.
- *QRS width*: normal width and morphology.
- *P waves*: present and constant morphology.
- *Relationship between P waves and QRS complexes*: each P wave is followed by a QRS complex and each QRS complex is preceded by a P wave; PR interval is prolonged 0.25s (7 small squares).

The ECG in Figure 8.2 displays first degree AV block. This is an interesting case. It was recorded in a 24-year-old lady who had presented to hospital with endocarditis. She subsequently developed an aortic root abscess which, due to it close proximity to the bundle of His, began to affect the conduction system, resulting in profound first degree AV block. The lady underwent surgical intervention for her endocarditis and was fitted with a permanent pacemaker because the bundle of His became necrosed.

## SECOND DEGREE AV BLOCK MOBITZ TYPE 1 (WENCKEBACK PHENOMENON)

Second degree AV block is where some but not all of the P waves are conducted to the ventricles (Resuscitation Council UK, 2006). There are two classifications: type I and type II (see below), both named after Woldemar Mobitz, an early twentieth century

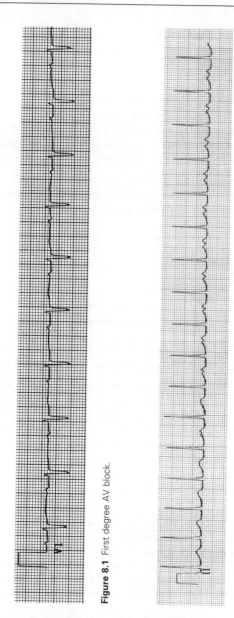

**Figure 8.1** First degree AV block.

**Figure 8.2** First degree AV block.

German internist. In the 1920s, he used an astute mathematical approach to classify second degree AV block into two types, subsequently referred to as Mobitz type I (Wenckeback) and Mobitz type II (Silverman *et al.*, 2004).

In 1849, before the availabilty of ECG recording, Karel Wenckebach, a Dutch anatomist, had investigated a woman who had consulted him about her irregular pulse (Upshaw & Silverman, 1999). He provided a description of irregular pulses due to partial blockage of AV conduction which created a progressive lengthening of conduction time in cardiac tissue (Wenckebach, 1899). This condition was later named the Wenckeback phenomenon.

Second degree AV block Mobitz type 1 is the commonest (90%) form of this degree of AV block (Jowett & Thompson, 1995). It can be caused by any condition that delays AV conduction (usually at the AV node), resulting in intermittent failure of transmission of the atrial impulse to the ventricles (Da Costa *et al.*, 2008). Causes include inferior myocardial infarction, electrolyte imbalance and drugs that suppress AV conduction, e.g. beta blockers, digoxin and calcium channel blockers (Docherty, 2003). It is sometimes benign (particularly during sleep) and is due to increased vagal tone (Bennett, 2006).

When associated with an inferior myocardial infarction, it usually has a gradual onset, progressing from first degree AV block over a period of hours and often leading on to third degree AV block, before reverting back to normal AV conduction after a further period of second degree AV block (Thompson, 1997). This sequence of events can be accelerated following right coronary reperfusion (Koren *et al.*, 1986).

It is characterised by a progressive prolongation of the PR interval until an impulse fails to be conducted to the ventricles, resulting in a dropped beat (QRS complex). This is then followed by a conducted impulse, with a shorter PR interval and a repetition of the cycle (Hampton, 2000). The number of dropped beats is variable. Sometimes gradual shortening of the RR interval is evident.

### Identifying features on the ECG

- *Electrical activity*: present.
- *QRS rate*: depending on the number of dropped beats, may be bradycardic.

- *QRS rhythm*: usually irregular (unless 2:1 conduction).
- *QRS width*: usually normal width and morphology.
- *P waves*: present and constant morphology, PP interval remains constant.
- *Relationship between P waves and QRS complexes*: not every P wave is followed by a QRS, but every QRS complex is preceded by a P wave; PR interval progressively lengthens until a QRS complex is dropped; RR interval progressively shortens.

**Effects on the patient**

The patient is rarely haemodynamically compromised, unless the ventricular rate is slow.

**Treatment**

Usually, the only active treatment required, apart from avoiding AV junctional blocking drugs, is close monitoring of the patient (Nolan *et al.*, 1998). If there is a risk of developing more severe AV block or asystole, treatment will be required (Resuscitation Council UK, 2006). If the ventricular rate is slow, atropine and, rarely, cardiac pacing may be required.

**Interpretation of Figure 8.3**

- *Electrical activity*: present.
- *QRS rate*: 50/min.
- *QRS rhythm*: irregular.
- *QRS width*: normal.
- *P waves*: present and constant morphology, PP interval remains constant.
- *Relationship between P waves and QRS complexes*: not every P wave is followed by a QRS, but every QRS complex is preceded by a P wave; PR interval progressively lengthens until a QRS complex is dropped.

The ECG in Figure 8.3 displays second degree AV block Mobitz type 1 (Wenckeback's phenomenon). It was seen in a patient with an acute inferior myocardial infarction and it followed a period of first degree AV block. On this occasion, because the ventricular rate was slow and the patient was haemodynamically compromised (BP 80/60 and complaining of dizziness), atropine 500 mcg IV was administered with effect.

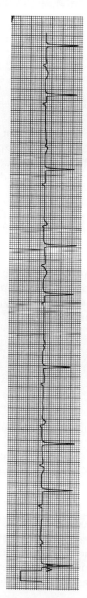

**Figure 8.3** Second degree AV block Mobitz type 1 (Wenckeback's phenomenon).

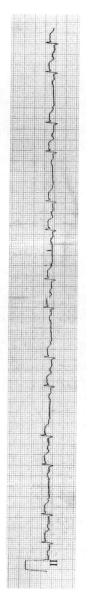

**Figure 8.4** Second degree AV block Mobitz type 1 (Wenckeback's phenomenon).

### Interpretation of Figure 8.4

- *Electrical activity*: present.
- *QRS rate*: 80/min.
- *QRS rhythm*: irregular.
- *QRS width*: normal.
- *P waves*: present and constant morphology, PP interval remains constant.
- *Relationship between P waves and QRS complexes*: not every P wave is followed by a QRS, but every QRS complex is preceded by a P wave; PR interval progressively lengthens until a QRS complex is dropped. Every third P wave is not conducted to the ventricles, i.e. 3:1 AV block.

The ECG in Figure 8.4 displays second degree AV block type 1 (Wenckeback's phenomenon). It was seen in a patient who had an acute inferior myocardial infarction 48 hours previously who developed chest pain again. The 12 lead ECG recorded in this patient suggests re-infarction. The ventricular rate was adequate and the patient was not haemodynamically compromised, so atropine was not required. However, the patient was reviewed by the cardiologist regarding the re-infarction.

### Interpretation of Figure 8.5

- *Electrical activity*: present.
- *QRS rate*: 85/min.
- *QRS rhythm*: irregular.
- *QRS width*: normal.
- *P waves*: present and constant morphology, PP interval remains constant.
- *Relationship between P waves and QRS complexes*: not every P wave is followed by a QRS, but every QRS complex is preceded by a P wave; PR interval progressively lengthens until a QRS complex is dropped.

The ECG in Figure 8.5 displays second degree AV block type 1 (Wenckeback's phenomenon). It was seen in a patient who presented with chest pain. The 12 lead ECG recorded in this patient suggests inferior lateral ischaemic changes. The ventricular rate was adequate and the patient was not haemodynamically

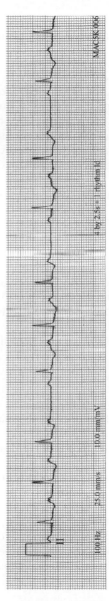

**Figure 8.5** Second degree AV block Mobitz type 1 (Wenckebach's phenomenon).

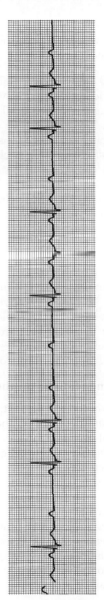

**Figure 8.6** Second degree AV block Mobitz type 2.

compromised, so atropine was not required. However, the patient was reviewed by the cardiologist and was referred for percutaneous coronary investigation (PCI).

## SECOND DEGREE AV BLOCK MOBITZ TYPE 2

Second degree AV block Mobitz type 2 is characterised by an intermittent failure of atrial impulse conduction to the ventricles (Bennett, 2006). It is not as common as second degree AV block type 1, but its implications are significantly more serious (Da Costa *et al.*, 2008). The block is usually at the level of the bundle branches, commonly resulting in a wide QRS complex (Da Costa *et al.*, 2008).

It is never a normal finding (Conover, 1992). It is often associated with advanced cardiac disease and often progresses to third degree AV block or asystole (Jowett & Thompson, 1995). If third degree AV block develops, it is often quite sudden and unexpected, with a slow ventricular escape rhythm and a marked deterioration in haemodynamic status (Brown *et al.*, 1969). Patients with anterior myocardial infarction who develop second degree AV block Mobitz type 2 have a poor prognosis (Nolan *et al.*, 1998).

In second degree AV block Mobitz type 2, the PR interval remains constant in the conducted beats, but some of the P waves are not followed by a QRS complex (Resuscitation Council UK, 2006), i.e. there are dropped beats.

### Identifying features on the ECG

- *Electrical activity*: present.
- *QRS rate*: depends on the number of dropped beats; may be normal or bradycardic.
- *QRS rhythm*: usually irregular due to dropped beats (unless 2:1 conduction).
- *QRS width*: usually wide (0.12 s/3 small squares or more) with bundle branch block pattern, may be normal width and morphology.
- *P waves*: present and constant morphology.
- *Relationship between P waves and QRS complexes*: not every P wave is followed by a QRS complex (dropped beats); every QRS complex is preceded by a P wave; PR interval constant, but may be prolonged.

### Effects on the patient

The patient is often haemodynamically compromised (Da Costa *et al.*, 2008). Progression to ventricular standstill and cardiac arrest is not uncommon.

### Treatment

Prophylactic temporary pacing is usually required (Nolan *et al.*, 1998).

### Interpretation of Figure 8.6

- *Electrical activity*: present.
- *QRS rate*: 50–60/min.
- *QRS rhythm*: irregular due to dropped beats.
- *QRS width*: normal width and morphology.
- *P waves*: present and constant morphology.
- *Relationship between P waves and QRS complexes*: not every P wave is followed by a QRS complex (dropped beats); every QRS complex is preceded by a P wave, PR interval constant.

The ECG in Figure 8.6 displays second degree AV block Mobitz type 2. This patient had been admitted with an acute anterior myocardial infarction. Although the patient was haemodynamically stable, there was a risk that the arrhythmia could degenerate into third degree AV block, or even ventricular standstill. Temporary cardiac pacing was required.

### Interpretation of Figure 8.7

- *Electrical activity*: present.
- *QRS rate*: 45/min.
- *QRS rhythm*: regular due to dropped beats.
- *QRS width*: normal width and morphology.
- *P waves*: present and constant morphology.
- *Relationship between P waves and QRS complexes*: not every P wave is followed by a QRS complex (dropped beats); every QRS complex is preceded by a P wave, PR interval constant.

The ECG in Figure 8.7 displays second degree AV block. From the ECG trace it is not possible to distinguish between second degree AV block types 1 and 2. However, ECG monitoring undertaken prior to recording the ECG trace showed isolated uncon-

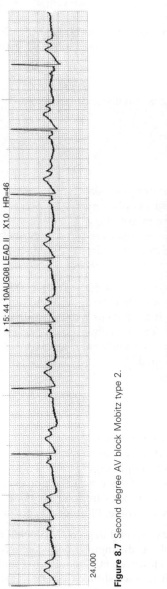

▶ 15: 44 10AUG08 LEAD II   X1.0   HR=46

24.000

**Figure 8.7** Second degree AV block Mobitz type 2.

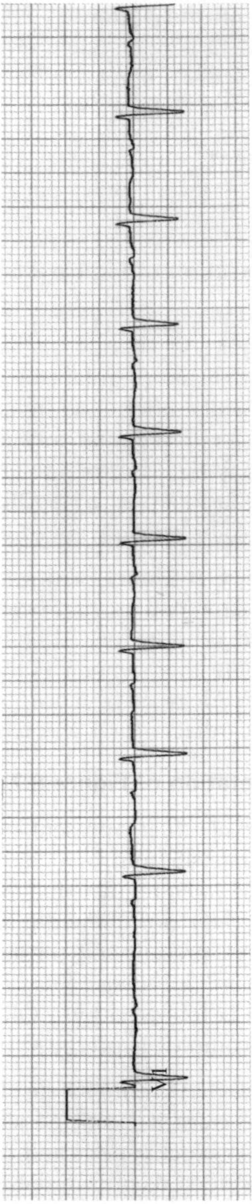

**Figure 8.8** Second degree AV block Mobitz type 2.

ducted P waves without PR interval prolongation, suggesting that the ECG trace must be second degree AV block type 2. This patient had been admitted with an acute myocardial infarction. His blood pressure was 80/50, he was cold and clammy and feeling lightheaded. Temporary cardiac pacing was required.

### Interpretation of Figure 8.8

- *Electrical activity*: present.
- *QRS rate*: 95/min.
- *QRS rhythm*: irregular due to dropped beat.
- *QRS width*: normal width and morphology.
- *P waves*: present and constant morphology.
- *Relationship between P waves and QRS complexes*: not every P wave is followed by a QRS complex (dropped beat); every QRS complex is preceded by a P wave, PR interval constant but prolonged.

The ECG in Figure 8.8 displays second degree AV block Mobitz type 2. This ECG was recorded in a 44-year-old lady undergoing an adenosine stress test (Myoview). One minute following the start of the adenosine infusion, the patient developed first degree AV block (prolonged PR interval) and then second degree AV block Mobitz type 2. She was feeling lightheaded. The adenosine infusion was immediately stopped and discontinued. She reverted back to sinus rhythm within two minutes. In this case, the AV conduction disturbances were caused by the adenosine.

### THIRD DEGREE AV BLOCK

Third degree AV block or complete AV block is where there is total failure of conduction between the atria and ventricle; it is characterised by AV dissociation – the P waves bear no relation to the QRS complexes and there is total independence of atrial and ventricular contractions (Da Costa *et al.*, 2008).

It can be an acute phenomenon, usually associated with a myocardial infarction, or may be chronic, usually caused by fibrosis of the bundle of His (Hampton, 2000). Other causes include cardiac surgery, endocarditis and drugs (Bennett, 2006). When associated with acute myocardial infarction, the pathophysiology and recommended treatment will depend on the site of the infarct (Nolan *et al.*, 1998).

When associated with an inferior myocardial infarction, it is normally caused by ischaemia or necrosis of the AV node, together with activation of the vagus nerve (Thompson, 1997). It develops slowly, being often preceded by first degree and then second degree AV block Mobitz type 1 (Wenckeback). It is generally well tolerated (Nolan *et al.*, 1998). The QRS complex is narrow, signifying a junctional escape rhythm which is usually reliable and of an adequate rate. Normal AV conduction usually resumes within 24 hours (Nolan *et al.*, 1998).

When associated with anterior myocardial infarction, it is frequently a sudden event, especially in patients who develop second degree AV block Mobitz type 2 or left bundle branch block (Nolan *et al.*, 1998). There is extensive necrosis of the septum, with damage to both the left and right bundle branches (Thompson, 1997). The QRS complex is wide, signifying a ventricular escape rhythm, unreliable and slow. The mortality rate in these patients is high (Nolan *et al.*, 1998).

Sometimes third degree AV block is a chronic phenomenon, particularly in the elderly. The patient may be admitted following a history of falls or blackouts: a diagnosis being made following a routine 12 lead ECG.

The rate and morphology of the escape rhythm is determined by the origin of the ventricular escape rhythm (Resuscitation Council UK, 2006). If the pacemaker site is situated in the AV node or proximal aspect of the bundle of His (more reliable), then the ventricular rate will be between 40–50 per minute (sometimes more) and the QRS width will be narrow; if the pacemaker site is in the distal His-Purkinje fibres or ventricular myocardium (less reliable), then the ventricular rate will be between 30–40 (sometimes less) and the QRS width will be wide – sudden ventricular standstill and cardiac arrest is possible (Resuscitation Council UK, 2006).

### Identifying features on the ECG

- *Electrical activity*: present.
- *QRS rate*: dependent upon the site of the subsidiary pacemaker; 40–60 if junctional, <40 if ventricular.
- *QRS rhythm*: regular.

- *QRS width*: may be normal (if junctional pacemaker), otherwise wide (0.12 s/3 small squares or more) with bundle branch block pattern (ventricular pacemaker).
- *P waves*: present and constant morphology, usually faster rate than the QRS complexes; absent if underlying rhythm is atrial fibrillation.
- *Relationship between P waves and QRS complexes*: no relationship with complete AV dissociation.

**Effects on the patient**
Some patients will have an adequate escape rhythm that will maintain their blood pressure, while others will be compromised, requiring urgent intervention. Generally, the effects on the patient will depend on the cause.

When associated with an anterior myocardial infarction, the patient is usually haemodynamically compromised. The risk of ventricular standstill and sudden cardiac arrest is high. If associated with an inferior myocardial infarction the patient may be haemodynamically stable. If chronic, the patient may present with a history of blackouts or falls.

**Treatment**
Again, this will depend on the cause. If associated with an inferior myocardial infarction, pacing will usually only be required if the ventricular rate is less than 40 or if the patient is haemodynamically compromised (Thompson, 1997). It may simply respond to I.V. atropine. If associated with an anterior myocardial infarction, a temporary and then often a permanent cardiac pacemaker will be required (ACC/AHA, 1991). External pacing is a recommended interim measure (Resuscitation Council UK, 2006). If chronic, a permanent pacemaker will usually be required.

**Interpretation of Figure 8.9**

- *Electrical activity*: present.
- *QRS rate*: 55/min.
- *QRS rhythm*: regular.
- *QRS width*: wide (0.12 s/3 small squares) and bizarre indicating a ventricular pacemaker.

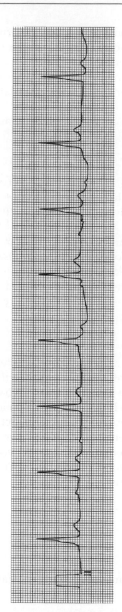

**Figure 8.9** Third degree AV block.

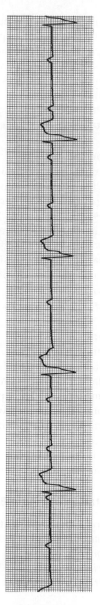

**Figure 8.10** Third degree AV block.

- *P waves*: present and constant morphology, rate 60/min; some appear on the T waves and some are hidden in the QRS complexes.
- *Relationship between P waves and QRS complexes*: AV dissociation.

The ECG in Figure 8.9 displays third degree AV block. This patient had been admitted with an inferior myocardial infarction. It was preceded by first degree AV block and then second degree AV block Mobitz type 1. It was only transient and it was well tolerated by the patient (BP 100/65). No intervention was required, except the administration of oxygen.

### Interpretation of Figure 8.10

- *Electrical activity*: present.
- *QRS rate*: 30/min
- *QRS rhythm*: regular.
- *QRS width*: wide (0.12 s/3 small squares) and bizarre indicating a ventricular pacemaker.
- *P waves*: present and constant morphology, rate 65/min; some appear on the T waves and some are hidden in the QRS complexes.
- *Relationship between P waves and QRS complexes*: AV dissociation.

The ECG in Figure 8.10 displays third degree AV block. This patient was admitted with a history suggestive of acute myocardial infarction. His blood pressure was unrecordable. He was unconscious. The patient required urgent cardiac pacing.

### Interpretation of Figure 8.11

- *Electrical activity*: present.
- *QRS rate*: 30/min.
- *QRS rhythm*: regular.
- *QRS width*: wide (0.12 s/3 small squares) and bizarre indicating a ventricular pacemaker.
- *P waves*: present and constant morphology, rate 65/min; some appear on the T waves and some are hidden in the QRS complexes.

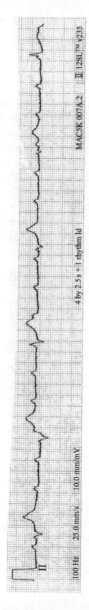

**Figure 8.11** Third degree AV block.

- *Relationship between P waves and QRS complexes*: AV dissociation.

The ECG in Figure 8.11 displays third degree AV block. It was recorded in an 82-year-old lady who had been admitted with a history of falls and blackouts for the previous four weeks, with a query over the cause. She was not haemodynamically compromised; her blood pressure was 166/58. She was reviewed by the cardiologist; she remained on an ECG monitor and a permanent pacemaker was arranged.

## CHAPTER SUMMARY

Cardiac arrhythmias with AV block can result from a conduction disturbance in the AV node, bundle of His or bundle branches. They are classified as first, second or third degree depending on whether impulse conduction to the ventricles is delayed, intermittently blocked or completely blocked (Bennett, 2006). Accurate interpretation is important because some are benign, whereas others can be life-threatening.

## REFERENCES

ACC/AHA (1991) Guidelines for implantation of cardiac pacemakers and anti-arrhythmic devices. A report of the ACC/AHA task force on assessment of diagnostic and therapeutic cardiovascular procedures (Committee on Pacemaker Implantation). *JACC*, **18**, 1–13.

Bennett DH (2006) *Cardiac Arrhythmias*, 6th edn. Butterworth Heinemann, Oxford.

Brown R, Hunt D, Sloman J (1969) The natural history of atrioventricular conduction defects in acute myocardial infarction. *American Heart Journal*, **78**, 460–466.

Conover M (1992) *Understanding Electrocardiography: Arrhythmias and the 12 Lead ECG*, 6th edn. Mosby-Year Book, St Louis.

Da Costa D, Brady W, Redhouse J (2008) Bradycardias and atrioventricular conduction block. In: Morris F, Brady W, Camm J (eds) *ABC of Clinical Electrocardiography*: Blackwell Publishing, Oxford.

Docherty B (2003) 12 lead ECG interpretation and chest pain management. *British Journal of Nursing*, **12** (21), 1248–1255.

Hampton J (2000) *The ECG Made Easy*, 5th edn. Churchill Livingstone, Edinburgh.

Jowett NI, Thompson DR (1995) *Comprehensive Coronary Care*, 2nd edn. Scutari Press, London.

Koren G, Weiss A, Ben-David T, *et al.* (1986) Bradycardia and hypotension following reperfusion with streptokinase (Bezold-Jarisch reflex): a sign of coronary thrombolysis and myocardial salvage. *American Heart Journal*, **112**, 468–471.

Nolan J, Greenwood J, Mackintosh A (1998) *Cardiac Emergencies: a Pocket Guide*. Butterworth Heinemann, Oxford.

Resuscitation Council UK (2006) *Advanced Life Support*, 5th edn. Resuscitation Council UK, London.

Silverman M, Upshaw C, Lange H (2004) Woldemar Mobitz and his 1924 classification of second-degree atrioventricular block. *Circulation*, **110**, 1162–1167.

Thompson P (1997) *Coronary Care Manual*. Churchill Livingstone, London.

Upshaw C, Silverman M (1999) The Wenckebach phenomenon: a salute and comment on the centennial of its original description. *Annals of Internal Medicine*, **130** (1), 58–63.

Wenckebach K (1899) *De Analyse van den onregelmatigen Pols. III. Over eenige Vormen van Allorythmie en Bradykardie*. Nederlandsch Tijdschrift voor Geneeskunde, Amsterdam, **2**, 1132.

# Cardiac Arrhythmias Associated with Cardiac Arrest

# 9

## INTRODUCTION

ECG rhythms associated with cardiac arrest are divided into two groups: shockable rhythms (ventricular fibrillation/pulseless ventricular tachycardia (VF/VT)) and non-shockable rhythms (asystole and pulseless electrical activity (PEA); the principal difference in the management of the two groups is the need for attempted defibrillation in those patients with VF/VT (Nolan et al., 2005).

Agonal rhythm (dying heart rhythm) will also be discussed. Ventricular tachycardia has been discussed in detail in Chapter 7 and will not be discussed again here.

The aim of this chapter is to recognise cardiac arrhythmias associated with cardiac arrest.

## LEARNING OUTCOMES

At the end of the chapter the reader will be able to state the characteristic ECG features of and outline the treatment for:

- ❏ Ventricular fibrillation.
- ❏ Asystole.
- ❏ Ventricular standstill.
- ❏ Pulseless electrical activity.
- ❏ Agonal rhythm.

## VENTRICULAR FIBRILLATION

*The cardiac pump is thrown out of gear, and the last of its vital energy is dissipated in a violent and prolonged turmoil of fruitless activity in the ventricular walls[e] … The normal beat is at once abolished,*

155

*and the ventricles are thrown into a tumultuous state of quick, irregular, twitching action; at the same time there is a great fall of blood-pressure. The ventricles become distended with blood, as the rapid quivering movement of their walls is wholly insufficient to expel their contents.*

*The muscular action partakes of the nature of an arrhythmic, inco-ordinated, and rapidly-repeated contraction of the various muscular bundles. Some bundles are in a state of contraction while other bundles are relaxed, and so, instead of a co-ordinated contraction leading to a definite narrowing of the ventricular cavity, there occurs an irregular and complicated arrhythmic oscillation of the ventricular walls which remain in a position of diastole. This condition is very persistent.*

(Reported in the British Medical Journal by
John McWilliam in 1889)

Sudden cardiac arrest (SCA) causes approximately 700,000 out-of-hospital deaths in Europe each year (Sans *et al.*, 1997). At the time of the first ECG analysis, about 40% of SCA victims have ventricular fibrillation (VF) (Cobb *et al.*, 2002; Rea *et al.*, 2004; Vaillancourt & Stiell, 2004). However, it is highly probable that many more sudden cardiac arrests are caused by VF (Handley *et al.*, 2005), but by the time ECG analysis has started, it has deteriorated into asystole (Waalewijn *et al.*, 2002). In hospital, VF is the presenting cardiac arrest arrhythmia in approximately 30% of arrests (Gwinnutt *et al.*, 2000).

An eminently treatable arrhythmia, the only effective treatment is early defibrillation and the likelihood of success is crucially time dependent (Resuscitation Council UK, 2006). Causes include ishaemic heart disease, heart failure, electrolyte imbalance, drugs, hypothermia and cardiomyopathy.

VF is characterised by chaotic, rapid depolarisation and repolarisation (Handley *et al.*, 2005). ECG features include a bizarre irregular waveform, apparently random in both amplitude and frequency, reflecting disorganised electrical activity in the myocardium. Initially the amplitude of the waveform is coarse. However, it will rapidly deteriorate into fine VF and then asystole, reflecting the depletion of myocardial high-energy phosphate stores (Mapin *et al.*, 1991).

## Identifying features on the ECG

- *Electrical activity*: present.
- *QRS rate*: no recognisable QRS complexes.
- *QRS rhythm*: no recognisable QRS complexes.
- *QRS width*: no recognisable QRS complexes.
- *P waves*: none recognisable.
- *Relationship between P waves and QRS complexes*: no recognisable P waves or QRS complexes present.

If electrical activity is present, but there are no recognisable complexes, the most likely diagnosis is ventricular fibrillation (Resuscitation Council UK, 2006).

## Effects on the patient

The patient will have a cardiac arrest.

## Treatment

The Resuscitation Council UK Advanced Life support algorithm details the treatment of VF/VT (see Figure 9.1). Early defibrillation is the definitive treatment for VT, the chances of success decline substantially (7–10%) for every minute it is delayed (Cobbe *et al.*, 1991). Adequate CPR can slow this decline (Larsen *et al.*, 1993). Forty-three per cent of patients who initially present with VF at the onset of a cardiac arrest survive to discharge (Gwinnutt *et al.*, 2000).

If VF/VT is confirmed, charge the defibrillator and deliver one shock (150–200 J biphasic or 360 J monophasic) (Nolan *et al.*, 2005). Then without reassessing the ECG or palpating a pulse, start or resume cardiopulmonary resuscitation (CPR) at a ratio of 30 compressions: 2 ventilations (Resuscitation Council UK, 2006). Further defibrillation is indicated if, after two minutes of CPR, VF/VT persists (see Figure 9.1). If VF/VT persists after three shocks, amiodarone 300 mg IV is recommended (Resuscitation Council UK, 2006).

Consider a precordial thump in a witnessed/monitored VF arrest if the defibrillator is not immediately at hand (Resuscitation Council UK, 2006); it will terminate VF in 2% of cases (Kerber & Robertson, 1996). It is most likely to be effective if delivered within 10 seconds of cardiac arrest (Kohl *et al.*, 2005).

Adult Advanced Life Support Algorithm

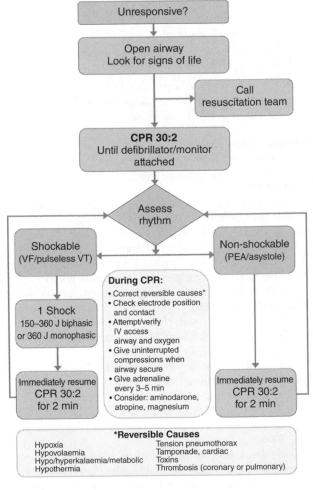

**Figure 9.1** Resuscitation Council UK advanced life support algorithm. Reproduced by kind permission from the Resuscitation Council UK.

**Interpretation of Figure 9.2**

- *Electrical activity*: present.
- *QRS rate*: no recognisable QRS complexes.
- *QRS rhythm*: no recognisable QRS complexes.
- *QRS width*: no recognisable QRS complexes.
- *P waves*: none recognisable.
- *Relationship between P waves and QRS complexes*: no recognisable P waves or QRS complexes present.

The ECG in Figure 9.2 displays VF. Treatment would be rapid defibrillation. CPR would be required while awaiting the defibrillator.

## ASYSTOLE

Asystole is the presenting rhythm in approximately 25% of in-hospital cardiac arrests (Gwinnutt *et al.*, 2000). In asystole, ventricular standstill is present owing to the suppression of all natural cardiac pacemakers.

Failure of sinus rhythm, under normal circumstances, will lead to the appearance of an escape rhythm maintained by a subsidiary pacemaker situated in either the AV junction (junctional rhythm) or ventricular myocardium (idioventricular rhythm). Myocardial disease, hypoxia, drugs and electrolyte imbalance can all suppress these escape rhythms.

It is most important to ensure the ECG trace is accurate. Other causes of a 'flat line' ECG trace include incorrect lead and ECG gain settings, and disconnected ECG leads (Jevon, 2002) (see Chapter 3). Sometimes, 'asystole' may be displayed on the monitor immediately following defibrillation, when monitoring using defibrillation paddles, regardless of the true ECG rhythm (Chamberlain, 1999). This is more common following multiple shocks and where there is high chest impedance (Bradbury *et al.*, 2000). If this phenomenon is encountered, the ECG leads should be used for ECG monitoring (Resuscitation Council UK, 2006).

**Identifying features on the ECG**

- *Electrical activity*: no electrical activity present.
- *QRS rate*: no electrical activity present.
- *QRS rhythm*: no electrical activity present.

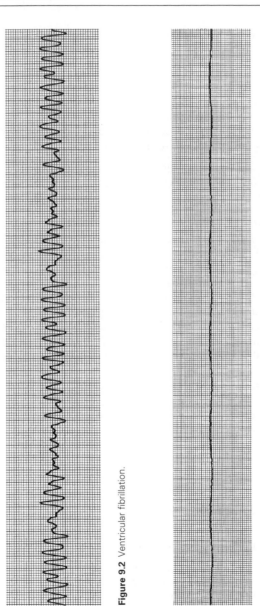

**Figure 9.2** Ventricular fibrillation.

**Figure 9.3** Asystole.

- *QRS width*: no electrical activity present.
- *P waves*: no electrical activity present.
- *Relationship between P waves and QRS complexes*: no electrical activity present.

**Effects on the patient**
The patient will have a cardiac arrest. The prognosis is very poor. Asystole is often terminal.

**Treatment**
Confirm cardiac arrest, check that the rhythm is indeed asystole and not, for example, ventricular fibrillation (ECG gain, lead connections, correct lead settings on the monitor) and, if indicated, start CPR.

The European Resuscitation Council guidelines for the management of asystole (non-VF/VT) (Latorre *et al.*, 2001) are depicted in Figure 9.1.

**Interpretation of Figure 9.3**

- *Electrical activity*: no electrical activity present.
- *QRS rate*: no electrical activity present.
- *QRS rhythm*: no electrical activity present.
- *QRS width*: no electrical activity present.
- *P waves*: no electrical activity present.
- *Relationship between P waves and QRS complexes*: no electrical activity present.

The ECG in Figure 9.3 displays probable asystole. Confirm cardiac arrest, check that the rhythm is indeed asystole and not, for example, ventricular fibrillation (ECG gain, lead connections, correct lead settings on the monitor) and, if indicated, start CPR.

VENTRICULAR STANDSTILL
Ventricular standstill is characterised by the presence of P waves and absent QRS complexes. One cause is that the sinus impulses are conducted to the ventricles, but the ventricles fail to respond to stimulation. Another cause is that they are not conducted to the ventricles because of the presence of complete AV block and an idioventricular rhythm fails to 'kick in'. Sometimes, ventricular standstill can occur quite suddenly if the patient is

already in second degree AV block Mobitz type 2 or third degree AV block.

### Identifying features on the ECG

- *Electrical activity*: present.
- *QRS rate*: no QRS complexes present.
- *QRS rhythm*: no QRS complexes present.
- *QRS width*: no QRS complexes present.
- *P waves*: present.
- *Relationship between P waves and QRS complexes*: no QRS complexes present.

### Effects on the patient

The patient will have a cardiac arrest.

### Treatment

Confirm cardiac arrest and start CPR following the non-shockable side of the ALS algorithm (see Figure 9.1). Emergency external pacing should be started. If capture is achieved and a pulse producing rhythm ensues, consider transvenous pacing.

### Interpretation of Figure 9.4

- *QRS rate*: no QRS complexes present.
- *QRS rhythm*: no QRS complexes present.
- *QRS complexes*: no QRS complexes present.
- *P waves*: present.
- *Relationship between P waves and QRS complexes*: no QRS complexes present.

The ECG in Figure 9.4 displays ventricular standstill. CPR would need to be started and external pacing requested.

### Interpretation of Figure 9.5

- *QRS rate*: intrinsic escaperhythm at 18/min and paced rhythm at 70/min.
- *QRS rhythm*: both paced and escape rhythm regular.
- *QRS width*: paced and escape rhythm QRS complexes wide.
- *P waves*: present.
- *Relationship between P waves and QRS complexes*: no relationship.

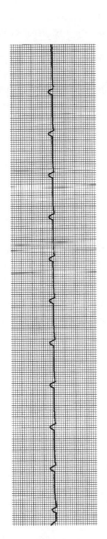

**Figure 9.4** Ventricular standstill.

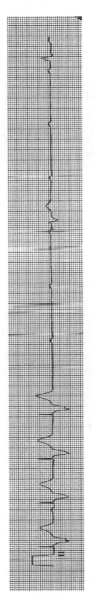

**Figure 9.5** Periods of ventricular standstill following ineffective transvenous pacing (due to malposition of pacing wire). Underlying rhythm is complete AV block with very slow ventricular escape at 18/min.

The ECG in Figure 9.5 displays ventricular standstill. This patient had a temporary transvenous cardiac pacemaker inserted for third degree AV block following an anterior myocardial infarction. Unfortunately it became ineffective due to malposition, resulting in ventricular standstill. External pacing was applied until the temporary transvenous pacing wire could be repositioned.

## PULSELESS ELECTRICAL ACTIVITY

Pulseless electrical activity (PEA) is the presenting rhythm in approximately 35% of in-hospital cardiac arrests (Gwinnutt *et al.*, 2000). PEA (formally called electromechanical dissociation or EMD) is a term used when there is no cardiac output, despite the presence of a normal (or near-normal) ECG. PEA can be classified as either primary or secondary.

Primary PEA is caused by a failure of excitation contraction coupling in the cardiac cells and causes a profound loss of cardiac output. Causes include massive myocardial infarction, poisoning and electrolyte imbalance. Secondary PEA is caused by a mechanical barrier to ventricular filling or ejection. Causes include cardiac tamponade, tension pneumothorax, pulmonary embolism and hypovolaemia. In all cases, treatment is directed at the cause.

### Identifying features on the ECG

The ECG trace displayed is normal or near-normal (Resuscitation Council UK, 2006). The patient could be in a state of cardiac arrest despite monitoring sinus rhythm.

### Effects on the patient

The patient will have a cardiac arrest.

### Treatment

Confirm cardiac arrest and start CPR. Treatment is aimed at identifying and treating the cause if possible. The Resuscitation Council UK algorithm for the management of pulseless electrical activity (non-VF/VT) is depicted in Figure 9.1.

## AGONAL RHYTHM

Agonal rhythm is characterised by slow, irregular, wide QRS complexes of varying morphology (Resuscitation Council UK,

2006). It is commonly described as the 'dying heart rhythm' and can be seen towards the end of an unsuccessful CPR attempt. True stimulation of the myocardium does not occur and it may continue for several minutes despite the patient being clinically dead (Meltzer *et al.*, 1983). The rate slows down until asystole ensues.

### Identifying features on the ECG

- *QRS rate*: usually very slow (<30/min).
- *QRS rhythm*: irregular.
- *QRS complexes*: very wide and bizarre.
- *P waves*: absent.
- *Relationship between P waves and QRS complexes*: unable to determine.

### Effects on the patient

The patient will already have had a cardiac arrest.

### Treatment

CPR will usually be stopped.

### Interpretation of Figure 9.6

- *QRS rate*: 25.
- *QRS rhythm*: regular.
- *QRS complexes*: very wide and bizarre.
- *P waves*: absent.
- *Relationship between P waves and QRS complexes*: no P waves present.

The ECG in Figure 9.6 displays agonal rhythm. It was recorded in a patient towards the end of an unsuccessful CPR attempt. The patient died.

### CHAPTER SUMMARY

Cardiac arrhythmias associated with cardiac arrest have been discussed in this chapter. These include ventricular fibrillation (VF), pulseless ventricular tachycardia (VT), asystole, ventricular standstill, pulseless electrical activity (formally called electromechanical dissociation or EMD) and agonal rhythm.

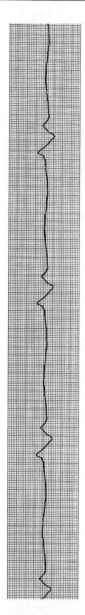

**Figure 9.6** Agonal rhythm.

## REFERENCES

Bradbury N, Hyde D, Nolan J (2000) Reliability of ECG monitoring with a gel pad/paddle combination after defibrillation. *Resuscitation*, **44**, 203–206.

Chamberlain D (1999) Spurious asystole with use of manual defibrillators. *British Medical Journal*, **319**, 1574.

Cobb L, Fahrenbruch C, Olsufka M, Copass M (2002) Changing incidence of out-of-hospital ventricular fibrillation, 1980–2000. *JAMA*, **288**, 3008–3013.

Cobbe S, Redmond M, Watson J, *et al.* (1991) Heartstart Scotland – initial experience of a national scheme for out of hospital defibrillation. *British Medical Journal*, **302**, 1517–1520.

Gwinnutt C, Columb M, Harris R (2000) Outcome after cardiac arrest in adults in UK hospitals: effect of the 1997 guidelines. *Resuscitation*, **47**, 125–135.

Handley A, Koster R, Monsieurs K, *et al.* (2005) European Resuscitation Council Guidelines for Resuscitation 2005 Section 2. Adult basic life support and use of automated external defibrillators. *Resuscitation*, **67S1**, S7–S23

Jevon P (2002) *Advanced Cardiac Life Support*. Butterworth Heinemann, Oxford.

Kerber R, Robertson C (1996) Transthoracic defibrillation. In: Paradis N, Halperin H, Nowak R (eds) *Cardiac Arrest: the Science and Practice of Resuscitation Medicine*. Williams & Wilkins, London.

Kohl P, King A, Boulin C (2005) Antiarrhythmic effects of acute mechanical stimulation. In: Kohl P, Sachs F, Franz MR (eds).*Cardiac Mechano-electric Feedback and Arrhythmias: From Pipette to Patient*. Elsevier Saunders, Philadelphia.

Larsen M, Eisenberg M, Cummins R, Hallstrom A (1993) Predicting survival from out-of-hospital cardiac arrest: a graphic model. *Annals of Emergency Medicine*, **22**, 85–91.

Latorre F, Nolan J, Robertson C, *et al.* (2001) European Resuscitation Council Guidelines 2000 for adult advanced life support. *Resuscitation*, **48**, 211–221.

McWilliam J (1889) Cardiac failure and sudden death. *British Medical Journal*, Jan, **5**, 6–8.

Mapin D, Brown C, Dzuonczyk R (1991) Frequency analysis of the human and swine electrocardiogram during ventricular fibrillation. *Resuscitation*, **22**, 85–91.

Meltzer LE, Pinneo R, Kitchell JR (1983) *Intensive Coronary Care: a Manual for Nurses*, 4th edn. Prentice Hall, London.

Nolan J, Deakin C, Soar J, *et al.* (2005) European Resuscitation Council Guidelines for Resuscitation 2005 Section 4. *Adult advanced life support Resuscitation*, **67S1**, S39–S86.

Rea T, Eisenberg M, Sinibaldi G, White RD (2004) Incidence of EMS-treated out-of-hospital cardiac arrest in the United States. *Resuscitation*, **63**,17–24.

Resuscitation Council UK (2006) *Advanced Life Support*, 5th edn. Resuscitation Council UK, London.

Sans S, Kesteloot H, Kromhout D (1997) The burden of cardiovascular diseases mortality in Europe. Task Force of the European Society of Cardiology on Cardiovascular Mortality and Morbidity Statistics in Europe. *Eur Heart J*, **18**,1231–1248.

Vaillancourt C, Stiell IG (2004) Cardiac arrest care and emergency medical services in Canada. *Can J Cardiol*, **20**,1081–1090.

Waalewijn R, Nijpels M, Tijssen J, Koster R (2002) Prevention of deterioration of ventricular fibrillation by basic life support during out-of-hospital cardiac arrest. *Resuscitation*, **54**, 31–36.

# Recording a 12 Lead ECG | **10**

## INTRODUCTION

An electrocardiograph (see Figure 10.1) is a machine that records the waveforms generated by the heart's electrical activity. An electrocardiogram (ECG) is a record or display of a person's heartbeat produced by an electrocardiograph (Soanes & Stevenson, 2006).

The recording of a 12 lead ECG must be undertaken meticulously. Care should be taken to ensure accuracy and standardisation: poor technique can lead to misinterpretation of the ECG, mistaken diagnosis, unnecessary investigations and mismanagement of the patient. To quote Marriott: 'heart disease of electrocardiographic origin should be avoided' (Wagner, 2000).

The aim of this chapter is to understand the principles of recording a 12 lead ECG.

## LEARNING OUTCOMES

At the end of the chapter the reader will be able to:

❑ List the common indications for recording a 12 lead ECG.
❑ Describe a procedure for recording a standard 12 lead ECG.
❑ Discuss how to ensure accuracy, quality and standardisation when recording a 12 lead ECG.
❑ Discuss what the standard 12 lead ECG records.

## COMMON INDICATIONS FOR RECORDING A 12 LEAD ECG

Common indications for recording a 12 lead ECG include:

• Chest pain.
• Myocardial infarction.
• Sometimes prior to a general anaesthetic.
• Cardiac arrhythmias.

- Palpitations.
- History of syncope.
- Following successful CPR.

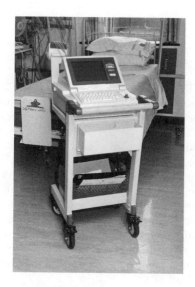

**Figure 10.1** Electrocardiograph or ECG machine.

## PROCEDURE FOR RECORDING A STANDARD 12 LEAD ECG

A suggested procedure for recording a standard 12 lead ECG is:

(1) Identify the patient.
(2) Explain the procedure to the patient.
(3) Assemble the equipment. It is important to ensure that the ECG cables are not twisted as this can cause interference (Metcalfe, 2000).
(4) Ensure the environment is warm and the patient is as relaxed as possible. This will help produce a clear, stable trace without interference.
(5) Ensure the patient is lying down in a comfortable position, ideally resting against a pillow at an angle of 45° with the head well supported (identical patient position should be

adopted as with previous 12 lead ECGs: this will help ensure standardisation). The inner aspects of the wrists should be close to, but not touching, the patient's waist.

(6) Prepare the skin if necessary. If wet gel electrodes are used, shaving and abrading the skin is not required. If solid gel electrodes are used, clean/ degrease and debride the skin and shave if necessary.

(7) Apply the electrodes (see Figure 10.2) and the limb leads:
   (a) red to the inner right wrist;
   (b) yellow to the inner left wrist;
   (c) black to the inner right leg, just above the ankle;
   (d) green to the inner left leg, just above the ankle.

(8) Apply the electrodes to the chest (see Figure 10.3a) and attach the chest leads:
   (a) V1 (white/red lead): fourth intercostal space, just to the right of the sternum;
   (b) V2 (white/yellow lead): fourth intercostal space, just to the left of the sternum;
   (c) V3 (white/green lead): midway between V2 and V4;
   (d) V4 (white/brown lead): fifth intercostal space, mid-clavicular line;
   (e) V5 (white/black lead): on anterior axillary line, on the same horizontal line as V4;
   (f) V6 (white/violet lead): mid-axillary line, on the same horizontal line as V4 and V5.

(9) Check the calibration signal on the ECG machine to ensure standardisation (Metcalfe, 2000).

(10) Ask the patient to lie still and breathe normally.

(11) Print out the ECG following the manufacturer's recommendations.

(12) Once an adequate 12 lead ECG has been recorded, disconnect the patient from the ECG machine. Clear equipment away and clean as necessary following the manufacturer's recommendations. Sometimes, electrodes are left on the patient if serial recordings are going to be required.

(13) Ensure the ECG is correctly labelled. Report and store the ECG in the correct patient's notes following local procedures.

(Jevon, 2007)

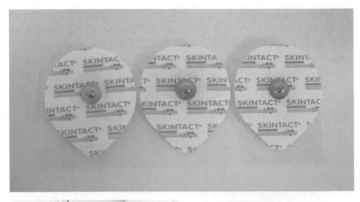

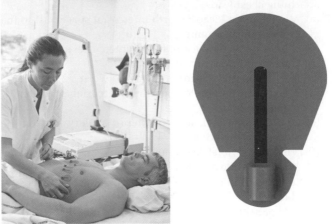

**Figure 10.2** ECG electrodes. Reproduced by kind permission of Ambu.

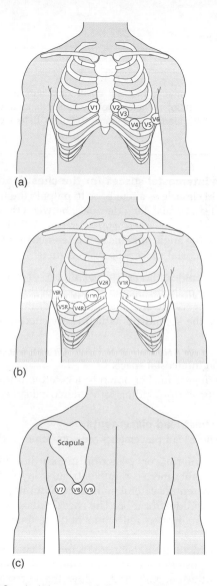

**Figure 10.3 (a)** Standard placement of chest leads. Reprinted from Morris F, *et al.*, *ABC of Clinical Electrocardiography*, 2nd edn, copyright 2008, with permission of Blackwell Publishing. **(b)** Alternative placement of chest leads to detect right ventricular infarction: right-sided chest leads. Reprinted from Morris F, *et al.*, *ABC of Clinical Electrocardiography*, 2nd edn, copyright 2008, with permission of Blackwell Publishing. **(c)** Alternative placement of chest leads to detect posterior infarction: posterior chest leads. Reprinted from Morris, F. *et al.*, *ABC of Clinical Electrocardiography*, 2nd edn, copyright 2008, with permission of Blackwell Publishing.

> Alternative placements of chest electrodes: right chest leads
> (see Figure 10.3b) to detect right ventricular infarction and
> posterior chest leads (see Figure 10.3c) to detect posterior
> infection.

### Locating the intercostal spaces for the chest leads

Using the right clavicle as a reference to palpate the first intercostal space can lead to mistaking the space between the clavicle and the first rib as the first intercostal space. It is therefore recommended to use the angle of Louis as a reference point for locating the second intercostal space. The procedure is:

(1) Palpate the angle of Louis (sternal angle) – it is at the junction between the manubrium and the body of the sternum.
(2) Slide the fingers towards the right side of the patient's chest and locate the second rib, which is attached to the angle of Louis.
(3) Slide the fingers down towards the patient's feet and locate the second intercostal space.
(4) Slide the fingers further down to locate the third and fourth ribs and the corresponding four intercostal spaces.

### Alternative chest lead placements

Alternative chest lead placements are sometimes indicated:

- *Right-sided*: inferior or posterior myocardial infarction, to ascertain whether there is right ventricular involvement (these patients may require careful management for hypotension and pain relief) and dextrocardia. The chest leads are labelled V3R to V6R and are in effect reflections of the left-sided chest leads V3 to V6.
- *Posterior*: particularly if there are reciprocal changes in V1–V2, suggesting posterior myocardial infarction. Chest leads are applied to the patient's back below the left scapula, corresponding to the same level as the fifth intercostal space, to view the posterior surface of the heart.
- *Higher or more lateral on the chest*: if the clinical history is suggestive of myocardial infarction, but the ECG is inconclusive.

## Labelling the 12 lead ECG

Labelling the 12 lead ECG should follow local protocols (often done electronically). All relevant information should be included, i.e. patient details (name, unit number, date of birth), date and time of recording, ECG serial number, together with any relevant information, e.g. if the patient was free from pain or complaining of chest pain during the recording, post-thrombolysis. The leads should be correctly labelled and deviations to the standard recording of a 12 lead ECG should be noted, e.g. right-sided chest leads, paper speed of 50 mm/s, different patient position.

## ENSURING ACCURACY, QUALITY AND STANDARDISATION WHEN RECORDING A 12 LEAD ECG

Many variables can influence the recording of a 12 lead ECG trace, without introducing unnecessary technical ones (Marriott, 1988). Deviations from the standard procedure for the recording of a 12 lead ECG can lead to misinterpretation and misdiagnosis. It is therefore important to ensure accuracy, quality and standardisation when recording a 12 lead ECG.

### Accuracy

Errors in electrode connection or placement are common (Jowett & Thompson, 1995). Slight displacement of the chest leads can produce considerable changes in the ECG pattern (Marriott, 1988). Interchanging limb leads could result in serious misinterpretation of the ECG, e.g. interchanged right arm and left leg leads produces a pattern mimicking inferior myocardial infarction with aVF resembling aVR.

### Quality

Poor electrode contact, patient movement and electrical interference, e.g. from infusion pumps by the bed, can cause a fuzzy appearance on the ECG trace. Efforts should be made to minimise interference, ensure good electrode contact and relax the patient. Other electrical devices should be moved away from the patient.

### Standardisation

- To help comparison of serial 12 lead ECGs, they should be recorded with the patient in the same position. If this is not

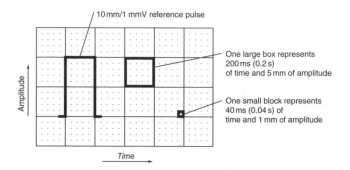

**Figure 10.4** Standard calibration. Reproduced by kind permission of Medtronic.

possible, e.g. if the patient has orthopnoea, a note to this effect should be made because the electrical axis of the heart (main direction of current flow) can be altered, which makes reviewing and comparing serial ECGs difficult (Wagner, 2000).

- Standard calibration is 1 mV vertical deflection on the ECG (see Figure 10.4). If calibration varies from recording to recording, ECG changes can sometimes be difficult to detect and the interpreter has to take into account inconsistencies in standardisation (Wagner, 2000).
- Standard paper speed is 25 mm/s.

NB Any deviations to the standard procedure for the recording of a 12 lead ECG should be highlighted on the ECG. This will help to avoid possible misinterpretation and misdiagnosis.

## WHAT THE STANDARD 12 LEAD ECG RECORDS

The heart generates electrical forces, which travel in multiple directions simultaneously. If the flow of current is recorded in several planes, a comprehensive view of this electrical activity can be obtained.

The standard 12 lead ECG records the electrical activity of the heart from 12 different viewpoints or leads ('leads' are viewpoints of the heart's electrical activity, they do not refer to the cables or wires which connect the patient to the monitor or ECG machine) by attaching 10 leads to the patient's limbs and chest.

### Limb leads

If leads are attached to the patient's right arm, left arm and left foot, the three major planes for detecting electrical activity can be recorded (a fourth lead, attached to the right leg serves as a neutral electrode and is not used for recording). A hypothetical triangle (Einthoven's triangle) is formed by these three axes, with the heart in the middle (see Figure 10.5).

## Frontal plane

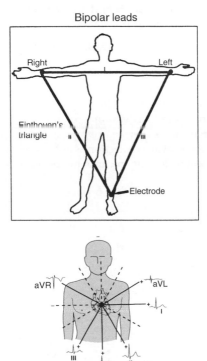

**Figure 10.5** Einthoven's triangle. Reproduced by kind permission of Philips Healthcare and Medtronic.

These three different views of the heart are designated standard leads I, II and III (Jowett & Thompson, 1995) and each records the difference in electrical forces between the two lead sites (Meltzer *et al.*, 1983), hence the term bipolar leads. This electrode placement also permits recording from three unipolar leads: aVR, aVL and aVF.

### Chest leads

The six chest leads view the heart in a horizontal plane from the front (anterior) and from the side (lateral) (see Figure 10.6).

### Standard placement of limb and chest leads and their relation to the surface of the heart

- Inferior surface of the heart: leads II, III, aVF.
- Anterior surface of the heart: leads V1, V2, V3, V4.
- Lateral surface of the heart: leads I, aVL, V5, V6.
- Septum: leads V2, V3.

### Configuration of the ECG waveform

Electrical current flows between two poles, a positive one and a negative one. An upward deflection will be recorded on the ECG when the current is flowing towards the positive pole; whereas a

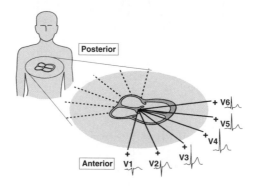

**Figure 10.6** Horizontal plane (chest leads). Reproduced by kind permission of Medtronic.

downward deflection will be recorded if the current is flowing away from the positive pole.

If an impulse is travelling towards a lead then the QRS complex in that lead will be predominantly positive, whereas if it is moving away from the lead it will be predominantly negative.

During depolarisation of the intraventricular septum, the impulse travels initially from left to right (see Figure 10.7). The impulse then travels down the bundle branches and Purkinje fibres resulting in multidirectional and simultaneous ventricular depolarisation (see Figure 10.7). In normal circumstances, the overall direction of depolarisation is towards the dominant mass of the left ventricle (see Figure 10.7). This results in:

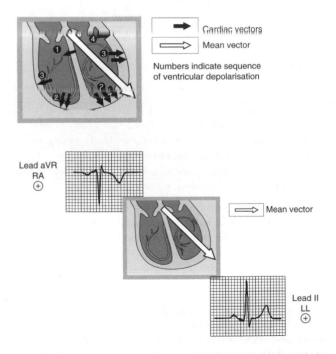

**Figure 10.7** Mean vector of electrical activity. Reproduced by kind permission of Medtronic.

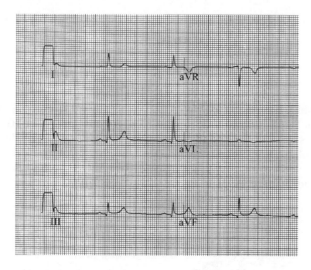

**Figure 10.8** Typical ECG configuration in the limb leads.

- Small Q waves and tall R waves in leads facing the left ventricle, e.g. leads II, V5, V6.
- Small R waves and deep S waves in leads facing the right ventricle, e.g. V1, V2 (see Figure 10.7).
- R and S waves of equal size when the wave of depolarisation is at right angles to the lead, e.g. aVL.

Consequently the configuration of the ECG waveform will depend upon the ECG lead being monitored. Figures 10.8 and 10.9 depict typical ECG configurations in the limb and chest leads respectively.

### CHAPTER SUMMARY
The 12 lead ECG is an essential diagnostic tool in the management of heart disease, in particular acute myocardial infarction. When recording a 12 lead ECG, care should be taken to ensure accuracy and standardisation in order to avoid possible misinterpretation of the ECG and mismanagement of the patient.

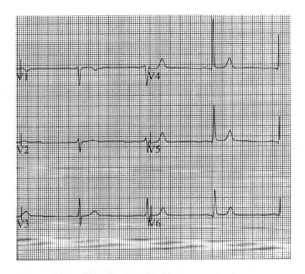

**Figure 10.9** Typical ECG configuration in the chest leads.

## REFERENCES

Jevon P (2007) Cardiac monitoring part 2: recording a 12 lead ECG. *Nursing Times*, **103** (2), 26–27.

Jowett NI, Thompson DR (1995) *Comprehensive Coronary Care*, 2nd edn. Scutari Press, London.

Marriott HJL (1988) *Practical Electrocardiography*, 8th edn. Williams & Wilkins, London.

Meltzer LE, Pinneo R, Kitchell JR (1983) *Intensive Coronary Care: a Manual for Nurses*, 4th edn. Prentice Hall, London.

Metcalfe H (2000) Recording a 12 lead electrocardiogram – 3. *Nursing Times*, **96** (22), 45–46.

Soanes C, Stevenson A (2006) *Oxford Dictionary of English*. Oxford University Press, Oxford.

Wagner G (2000) *Practical Electrocardiography*. Williams & Wilkins, London.

# 11 | Interpreting a 12 Lead ECG

## INTRODUCTION

The 12 lead ECG is an essential diagnostic tool in the management of heart disease. In particular, with the advent of thrombolytic therapy, the 12 lead ECG plays an important role in the early diagnosis of acute myocardial infarction. In addition, it can provide detailed and useful information when interpreting cardiac arrhythmias. When interpreting it in light of the clinical history, the ECG can be invaluable in aiding selection of the most appropriate management (Channer & Morris, 2008).

The aim of this chapter is to understand the principles of interpreting a 12 lead ECG.

## LEARNING OUTCOMES

At the end of the chapter the reader will be able to:

❑ Describe a systematic approach to the interpretation of a 12 lead ECG.
❑ Discuss the ECG features associated with myocardial infarction.
❑ Discuss the ECG features associated with myocardial ischaemia.
❑ Discuss the ECG changes associated with bundle branch block.
❑ Interpret a selection of 12 lead ECGs.

## SYSTEMATIC APPROACH TO THE INTERPRETATION OF A 12 LEAD ECG

A systematic approach to the interpretation of a 12 lead ECG involves examining/checking:

- Patient and ECG details.
- Calibration.

- P waves.
- PR interval.
- QRS rate.
- QRS rhythm.
- QRS complexes.
- T waves.
- ST segment.
- QT interval.
- U waves.
- Relationship between the P waves and QRS complexes.
- The rhythm.
- Electrical axis.
- Previous ECGs.

### Patient and ECG details

Check the patient details: name, hospital number, etc. Also check the ECG details, including date and time of recording and whether there were any deviations to the standard approach to the recording of a 12 lead ECG.

### Calibration

Check the calibration of the ECG (see Figure 10.5 in Chapter 10).

### P waves

Establish whether P waves are present. If they are present determine the rate and whether their morphology is normal and constant. As atrial activation spreads across the atria in an inferior direction towards the AV junction, P waves are usually upright in leads facing the inferior surface of the heart (leads II, III and aVF) and inverted in aVR which faces the superior surface.

Changes in P wave morphology imply a different pacemaker focus for the impulse. Retrograde activation through the AV junction (junctional or ventricular arrhythmias) usually results in the P waves being inverted in leads II, III and aVF (atrial depolarisation opposite direction to normal).

The amplitude should not exceed 0.3 mV (3 small squares), the width should not exceed 0.11 s (2.75 small squares) and the shape should be round, not notched or pointed. When examining P waves it is important to look for the following abnormalities:

- *Increased amplitude* (>0.3 mV): usually indicative of atrial hypertrophy or dilation. Often associated with hypertension or AV valve disease.
- *Increased duration* (>0.11 s): usually indicative of left atrial enlargement.
- *Inversion in leads when normally upright*: inverted P waves in leads I and II are indicative of the spread of the impulse across the atria in an unorthodox way, e.g. atrial premature beat (APB), junctional premature beat (JPB).
- *Notching*: left atrial enlargement, sometimes referred to as P mitrale.
- *Peak complex*: tall, pointed P waves, more noticeable in lead III than in lead I, resulting from right atrial overload, sometimes referred to as P pulmonale.
- *Diphasicity*: when the second part of the P wave is significantly negative in lead III or V1, it is an important sign of left atrial enlargement.

Sometimes, it may be difficult to establish whether P waves are present because they are partly or totally obscured by the QRS complexes or T waves, e.g. in sinus tachycardia P waves may merge with the preceding T waves.

In SA block and sinus arrest, P waves will be absent. In atrial fibrillation, no P waves can be identified, just a fluctuating baseline. In atrial flutter, P waves are replaced by regular sawtooth flutter waves, at a rate of approximately 300/min.

**PR interval**

Calculate the PR interval. It represents the time taken for the impulse to travel from the SA node to the ventricles. It is measured from the beginning of the P wave to the beginning of the QRS complex. The normal PR interval is 0.12–0.20 s (3–5 small squares). It varies with heart rate: the faster the heart rate, the shorter the interval.

A prolonged PR interval (>0.20 s) is indicative of AV block. Sometimes it is a normal variation. A shortened PR interval

(<0.12s) is associated with an AV junctional pacemaker or the presence of an accessory pathway, e.g. Wolff-Parkinson-White syndrome.

## QRS rate

Estimate the QRS rate by counting the number of large squares between two adjacent QRS complexes and dividing it into 300 (caution if the QRS rate is irregular). For example, the QRS rate in Figure 3.2 in Chapter 3 is about 75/min (300/4).

An alternative method is to count the number of QRS complexes in a defined number of seconds and then calculate the rate per minute. For example, if there are 12 QRS complexes in a 10s strip; ventricular rate is 72/min (12 × 6).

- Normal QRS rate: 60–100/min.
- Slow QRS rate (bradycardia): <60/min.
- Fast QRS rate (tachycardia): >100/min.

NB A pulse rate of 50/min may be 'normal' in some patients and one of 70/min may be abnormally slow in other patients.

## QRS rhythm

Ascertain whether the QRS rhythm is regular or irregular. Using the rhythm strip displayed on the ECG, carefully compare RR intervals. Callipers may help.

Alternatively, plot two QRS complexes on a piece of paper. Then move the paper to other sections on the rhythm strip and ascertain whether the marks are aligned exactly with other pairs of QRS complexes (regular QRS rhythm) or not (irregular QRS rhythm) (see Figure 3.4 on page 47).

If the QRS rhythm is found to be irregular, determine whether it is totally irregular or whether there is a cyclical variation in the RR intervals (Resuscitation Council UK, 2006).

A totally irregular QRS rhythm most likely indicates atrial fibrillation, particularly if the morphology of the QRS complexes remains constant. If there is a cyclical pattern to the irregularity of the RR intervals, examine the relationship between the P waves and QRS complexes (see below). The presence of ectopics can render an otherwise regular QRS rhythm irregular. Determine whether they are atrial, junctional or ventricular.

### QRS complexes

Examine the morphology of the QRS complexes. The QRS complex represents the spread of the impulse through the ventricles and is labelled as follows:

- Q wave: if the first deflection of the complex is negative or downward.
- R wave: the first positive or upright deflection.
- S wave: negative deflection following an R wave.
- R1: if there is a second positive deflection.
- S1: if there is a second negative deflection.

Lower case and capital letters are used to describe the relative sizes of the QRS components. When examining the morphology of the QRS complexes, measure the width and amplitude and examine any Q waves.

### *Width*

Normal width is <0.12 s/3 small squares. A QRS width of 0.12 s/3 small squares or more is indicative of abnormal intraventricular conduction, either bundle branch block or a ventricular arrhythmia.

If the patient has a tachyarrhythmia with a wide QRS complex, it is important to establish whether it is supraventricular or ventricular in origin. Supraventricular tachycardia with aberration (i.e. impulses are conducted to the ventricles with bundle branch block resulting in wide QRS complexes) can mimic ventricular tachycardia. Most wide complex tachycardias are ventricular in origin. According to Wagner (2000), the following ECG features favour ventricular origin:

- R or qR (rabbit ear) in V1.
- rS or QS in V6.
- All QRS complexes in the chest leads either positive or negative (concordance).
- Extreme axis deviation (90° to 180°) – positive aVR.
- QRS complex > 0.14 s/3.5 small squares.
- Presence of fusion beats and/or capture beats.
- AV dissociation.

According to Wagner (2000), the following ECG features favour aberrant conduction:

- rsR morphology in V1.
- qRs morphology in V6.
- QRS morphology identical to pre-existing bundle branch block.
- If there is right bundle branch block and the initial QRS deflection is identical to that with the normal beats.

### Amplitude (voltage)

The total amplitude, i.e. above and below the isoelectric line, should be greater than 0.5 mV (5 small squares) in the standard limb leads. Abnormally low voltage may be seen in pericardial effusion, myxoedema and widespread myocardial damage. The distance the recording leads are away from the heart can also influence the voltage – chest size, chest wall thickness, etc. should be taken into account when examining the amplitude.

Ventricular hypertrophy will result in increased electrical activity and an increase in height of the QRS complex. In right ventricular hypertrophy, the lead facing the right ventricle (V1) displays dominant R waves at least 0.5 mV (5 small squares) tall instead of the usual dominant S waves (Julian & Cowan, 1993). In left ventricular hypertrophy, the leads facing the left ventricle (V5 and V6) display tall R waves > 2.5 mV (25 small squares) and the lead facing the right ventricle (V1) displays deep S waves.

### Q waves

Small narrow Q waves are normal in leads facing the left ventricle, i.e. lead I, aVL, aVF, V5 and V6. Wide (>0.04 s/1 small square) and deep (>0.2 mV/2 small squares) Q waves are indicative of myocardial infarction (Hampton, 2000). The presence of Q waves in lead III is sometimes a normal finding.

### T waves

Examine the T waves. They represent repolarisation of the ventricles. Note the direction, shape and height. They are normally upright in leads I, II and V3–V6, inverted in aVR and variable in the other leads. They are normally slightly rounded and asymmetrical. Their height should not be > 0.5 mV (5 small squares) in the standard leads or >1.0 mV (10 small squares) in the chest leads.

Sharply pointed T waves are suggestive of myocardial infarction or hyperkalaemia. Notched T waves are sometimes found in pericarditis. Inverted T waves can be associated with myocardial ischaemia, digoxin toxicity and ventricular hypertrophy.

The T wave morphology can be affected by myocardial ischaemia in a variety of different ways: tall, flattened, inverted or biphasic (Channer & Morris, 2008). In ventricular hypertrophy the T waves are inverted and asymmetrical (Julian & Cowan, 1993). In left ventricular hypertrophy, the T waves are inverted in the left ventricular leads, i.e. leads II, aVL, V5 and V6; in right ventricular hypertrophy, the T waves are inverted in the right ventricular leads, i.e. V2 and V3 (Hampton, 2000).

## ST segment

Examine the ST segment. It represents the period following ventricular depolarisation (end of QRS complex) to the beginning of ventricular repolarisation (beginning of the T wave). It is usually isoelectric. Note the level of the ST segment in relation to the baseline (elevation or depression) and also its shape.

Elevation or depression is indicative of an abnormality in the onset of ventricular muscle recovery. Elevation >0.1 mV (1 small square) in the limb leads and >0.2 mV (2 small squares) in the chest leads is abnormal. The commonest cause of ST segment elevation is myocardial infarction. Widespread (and not localised) ST segment elevation (concave upwards) is characteristic of pericarditis. ST segment elevation is sometimes a normal finding in healthy young black men (Marriott, 1988).

The ST segment shape should gently curve into the T wave. Depression > 0.5 mV (0.5 small square) is abnormal (Julian & Cowan, 1993). Horizontal depression of the ST segment, together with an upright T wave, is usually indicative of myocardial ischaemia (Hampton, 2000). In digoxin toxicity, the ST segment is down-sloping or sagging (Channer & Morris, 2008), particularly prominent in leads II and III.

## QT interval

Calculate the QT interval. It represents the total duration of ventricular depolarisation and repolarisation. It is measured from the beginning of the QRS complex to the end of the T wave. It varies with heart rate, sex (longer in women) and age. The normal QT interval is usually less than half of the preceding RR interval (Marriott, 1988) and the upper limit of normal is 0.40 s/2 large squares (Hampton, 2000).

A prolonged QT interval indicates that ventricular repolarisation is delayed, which could result in the development of tachyarrhythmias. Causes of a prolonged QT interval include genetic, drugs, hypothermia and electrolyte imbalance.

**U waves**

U waves are low voltage waves that may be seen following the T waves. Their source is uncertain (Marriott, 1988). They share the same polarity as the T waves and are best viewed in V3. They are more prominent in hypokalaemia.

**Relationship between the P waves and QRS complexes**

Establish whether the P waves and QRS complexes are associated with to each other. Ascertain whether each P wave is followed by a QRS complex and each QRS complex is preceded by a P wave.

If the PR interval is constant, atrial and ventricular activity is likely to be associated. If the PR interval is variable, establish whether atrial and ventricular activity is associated or dissociated. Map out the P waves and QRS complexes and examine their relationship. Look for any recognisable patterns, the presence of dropped beats and PR intervals that vary in a repeated fashion (Resuscitation Council UK, 2006).

AV dissociation is when the atria and ventricles are depolarised by two different sources. It is seen, for example, in third degree (complete) AV block and sometimes in ventricular tachycardia. It is not a diagnosis in itself, but a clinical feature identified on the ECG of a cardiac arrhythmia.

**Electrical axis**

In order to depolarise every cardiac cell, the electrical impulses must travel in many different directions through the myocardium. These different directions of current flow collectively determine the electrical summation vector or axis during depolarisation and systole (Paul & Hebra, 1998). Normally, the axis is down and to the patient's left, reflecting the impulse direction

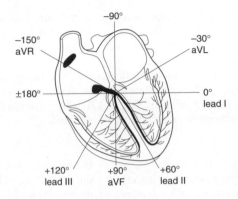

**Figure 11.1** Hexaxial reference system. Reproduced by kind permission of Williams & Wilkins.

down from the SA node, through the AV junction and down to and through the ventricles (see Figure 10.8 in Chapter 10).

For simplification, Marriott (1988) defines a normal axis as between 0° and 90°, right axis deviation as between 90° and 180°, and left axis deviation as between 0° and −90° (see Figure 11.1).

There are several methods that can be used to calculate the cardiac axis; some are more confusing than others. Some basic principles to consider when calculating the electrical axis are as follows:

- The lead with the largest positive QRS deflection is the closest of the six limb leads towards which the electrical summation vector or axis travels.
- The lead with the largest negative QRS deflection is the furthest of the six limb leads away from which the electrical summation vector or axis travels.
- The electrical axis points towards leads whose R waves are larger than the S waves.
- The electrical axis points away from leads whose R waves are smaller than the S waves.
- The electrical axis is at right angles to the lead with equally sized R and S waves.

Houghton & Gray (2003) suggest the following quick and simple technique for working out the cardiac axis. Examine leads I and II. If the QRS complex is:

- Predominantly positive in both leads I and II, the axis is normal.
- Predominantly positive in lead I but predominantly negative in lead II, there is left axis deviation.
- Predominantly negative in lead I, but predominantly positive in lead II, there is right axis deviation.

(For most practical purposes, it is not necessary to determine the exact axis of the heart.)

A useful aide-memoire is:

- If lead I is predominantly positive and lead III is predominantly negative, they will be pointing away from each other, i.e. they have *left* each other – left axis deviation.
- If lead I is predominantly negative and lead III is predominantly positive, they will be pointing towards each other, i.e. they are *right* for each other – right axis deviation.

Causes of left axis deviation include:

- Left bundle branch block.
- Left anterior fascicular block.
- Ventricular arrhythmias.

Causes of right axis deviation include:

- Right bundle branch block.
- Left posterior fascicular block.
- Ventricular arrhythmias.

## ECG CHANGES ASSOCIATED WITH MYOCARDIAL INFARCTION

Over 80% of patients with acute myocardial infarction present with an abnormal ECG (Jowett & Thompson, 1995). However, less than 50% of patients initially present with typical and diagnostic ECG changes (Channer & Morris, 2008). Sometimes the ECG may be normal or inconclusive. Nevertheless, despite some limitations, the ECG is probably still the best way of diagnosing myocardial infarction (Timmis, 1990).

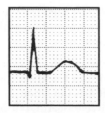

**Figure 11.2** Normal QRST complex. Reproduced by kind permission of Ambu.

Daily (often subtle) ECG changes can be of major value in the diagnosis of myocardial infarction, especially when they are interpreted with the knowledge of the clinical history and serum enzyme changes (Jowett & Thompson, 1995). Approximately 10% of patients with a proven myocardial infarction (clinical history and cardiac enzyme rises) fail to develop ST segment elevation or depression (Morris & Brady, 2008).

### Within minutes of myocardial infarction

Within minutes of myocardial infarction, the normal QRS complex (see Figure 11.2) with a tall R wave and a positive T wave, changes. The earliest signs are subtle: T waves over the affected area become more pronounced, symmetrical and pointed. These T waves, often referred to as 'hyperacute T waves', are more evident in the anterior leads and are more easily identified if an old 12 lead ECG is available for comparison (Morris & Brady, 2008).

These T wave changes are quickly followed by ST segment elevation (see Figure 11.3), which is often seen in leads facing the affected area of the myocardium. It is caused by damaged, but not necrosed, myocardial tissue. It can occur within minutes of the onset of chest pain and is a characteristic ECG change used as a criterion for the administration of thrombolytic therapy (Colquhoun, 1993).

### Hours to days following myocardial infarction

Hours to days following the event, in the leads facing the affected area, the R waves become smaller. Wide (>0.04 s or 1 small square)

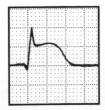

**Figure 11.3** ST segment elevation. Reproduced by kind permission of Ambu.

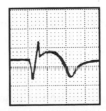

**Figure 11.4** ST segment begins to subside and T waves become increasingly negative. Reproduced by kind permission of Ambu.

and deep (>0.2 mV or 2 small squares) Q waves develop (Hampton, 2000). In addition, the ST elevation begins to subside and T waves become increasingly negative (Figure 11.4).

The presence of deep and broad Q waves indicates there is necrosed myocardial tissue in the heart which the leads face. The Q waves actually represent electrical activity in the opposite ventricular wall, which the leads view through an electrical window created by the necrosed (electrically inactive) myocardial tissue.

### Days to weeks following myocardial infarction

Days to weeks later, the ST segment returns to the baseline and the T waves become more inverted and symmetrical (see Figure 11.5). Sometimes the R wave completely disappears.

Although most Q waves persist following a myocardial infarction, up to 15% can regress within 18 months with some ECGs returning to normal after three years (Surawicz *et al.*, 1978).

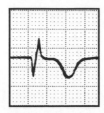

**Figure 11.5** Q waves and inverted T waves. Reproduced by kind permission of Ambu.

### Localising the myocardial infarction from the ECG

The characteristic changes seen in myocardial infarction are seen in the leads that record from the affected area. Familiarity with the areas of the myocardium represented by each of the ECG leads will enable not only the localisation of the infarction but also the extent of it. Common sites of infarction and the affected leads (Colquhoun, 1993) are summarised as follows:

- Inferior myocardial infarction: leads II, III, aVF.
- Lateral myocardial infarction: leads I, aVL, V5, V6.
- Anteroseptal myocardial infarction: V1, V2, V3, V4.
- Anterolateral myocardial infarction: I, aVL, V4, V5, V6.

Right ventricular myocardial infarction, which is associated with 40% of inferior myocardial infarctions, is often overlooked because the standard 12 lead ECG does not provide a good indication of right ventricular damage (Morris & Brady, 2008). The presence of ST elevation in V1 does suggest right ventricular damage. However, right-sided chest leads (see Figure 10.3b on page 173) are more sensitive and these should be recorded as soon as possible. Subsequent management may need to be modified if the infarction involves the right ventricle.

Posterior myocardial infarction is often missed because the standard 12 lead ECG does not include the posterior leads. ECG changes can be seen indirectly in leads V1–V3 which face the endocardial surface of the posterior wall of the left ventricle: the 'mirror image' includes tall R waves, ST depression and upright T waves (Morris & Brady, 2008). Posterior wall chest leads (see

Figure 10.3c on page 173) should be recorded to help confirm diagnosis.

### Q wave and non-Q wave infarctions

Q wave infarctions are commonly termed transmural or full-thickness infarctions. Non-Q wave infarctions are commonly termed not full-thickness or subendocardial infarctions. However, this pathology is often not correct (Hampton, 2000).

In an extensive myocardial infarction, Q waves are a permanent sign of necrosis. However, when the myocardial infarction is more localised, the scar tissue may contract during the healing process, reducing the size of the electrically inert area resulting in the disappearance of the Q waves (Morris & Brady, 2008).

### Reciprocal changes

ST depression in leads remote from the site of the infarct are referred to as reciprocal changes. They are a highly sensitive indicator of acute myocardial infarction (Morris & Brady, 2008). They may be seen in leads that do not directly view the affected area of myocardium (they reflect a mirror image of their opposite leads). In Figure 11.6, ST elevation is evident in the inferior leads with reciprocal changes in the lateral leads. The depressed ST segments are typically horizontal or downsloping.

Reciprocal changes are seen in approximately 70% of inferior and 30% of anterior myocardial infarctions (Morris & Brady, 2008). Reciprocal changes in the anterior chest leads V1–V3 are sometimes evident in a posterior myocardial infarction. The presence of reciprocal changes is particularly useful when there is doubt about the clinical significance of ST elevation (Morris & Brady, 2008).

### Diagnosing myocardial infarction in the presence of left bundle branch block

Diagnosing myocardial infarction in the presence of left bundle branch block can be very difficult. Q waves, ST segment and T wave changes can be obscured.

### ECG examples of myocardial infarction

The ECG in Figure 11.6 displays the characteristic ECG changes associated with acute inferior myocardial infarction. ST elevation

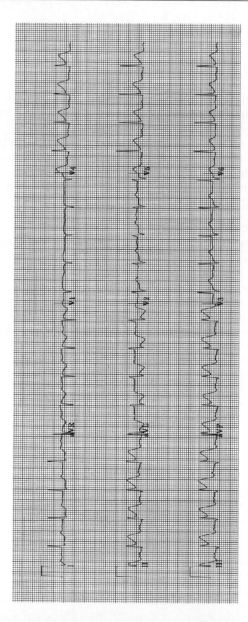

**Figure 11.6** Acute inferior myocardial infarction.

can clearly be seen in leads II, III and aVF. Reciprocal changes can be seen, most markedly in lead aVL. Subsequent ECGs will probably indicate lateral involvement as well, i.e. inferolateral myocardial infarction. The ECG in Figure 11.7, recorded with right-sided chest leads, displays right ventricular involvement. This patient was admitted with a one-hour history of crushing central chest pain. The ECG changes are typical of an acute myocardial infarction.

The ECG in Figure 11.8 displays the characteristic ECG changes associated with inferior myocardial infarction. There is ST elevation in the inferior leads (II, III and aVF). However, the T waves in these leads are beginning to become negative. This, with the development of Q waves in the inferior leads, is suggestive that the infarct is not acute. This patient was admitted with a 24-hour history of central chest pain.

The ECG in Figure 11.9 displays the characteristic ECG changes associated with posterior myocardial infarction. Tall R waves and ST depression in the anterior leads V1 and V2 and reciprocal changes in the lateral leads I and aVL would suggest this diagnosis. Posterior wall chest leads would be required to help confirm the diagnosis of a posterior myocardial infarction.

The ECG in Figure 11.10 displays the characteristic ECG changes associated with an anteroseptal or septal myocardial infarction. There is ST elevation in leads aVL and V1–V4. In addition, there is right bundle branch block and left anterior fascicular block (bifascicular block), a complication of septal infarction. Regarding the right bundle branch block the familiar rSR morphology has been replaced with QR morphology due to the infarction.

The ECG in Figure 11.11 displays the characteristic ECG changes associated with an anteroseptal myocardial infarction. The abnormally tall and peaked T waves in leads V1–V4 are very suggestive of this. These ECG changes are hyperacute and are occasionally seen in the septal chest leads. This patient was admitted by his GP with a one-hour history of chest pain.

## ECG CHANGES ASSOCIATED WITH MYOCARDIAL ISCHAEMIA

Myocardial ischaemia can cause changes in the ST segment and T wave but not the QRS complex (except if it causes bundle

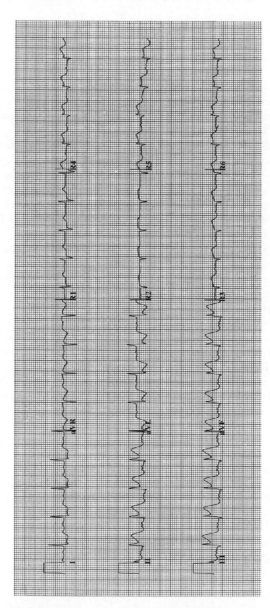

**Figure 11.7** Acute inferior myocardial infarction with right-sided chest leads indicating right ventricular involvement.

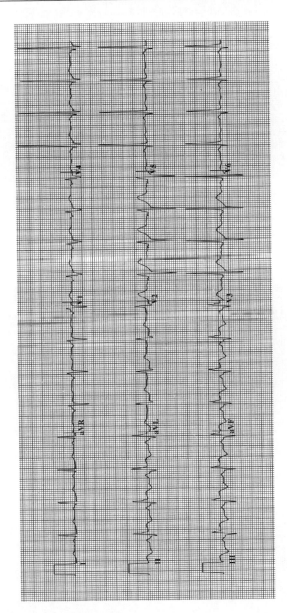

**Figure 11.8** Inferior myocardial infarction.

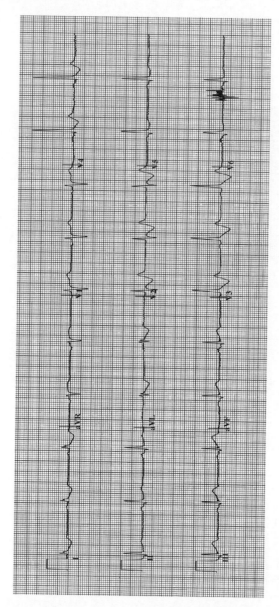

**Figure 11.9** Possible posterior myocardial infarction.

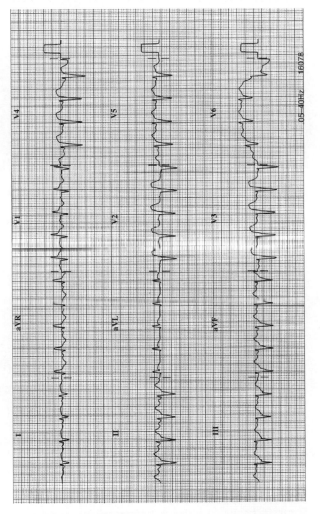

**Figure 11.10** Anteroseptal or septal myocardial infarction with bifascicular block.

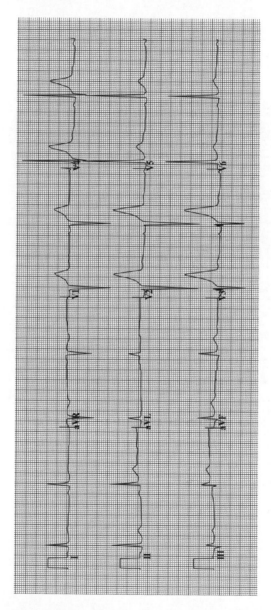

**Figure 11.11** Anteroseptal or septal myocardial infarction.

branch block) (Channer & Morris, 2008). Ischaemic changes associated with chest pain, but in the absence of myocardial infarction, are prognostically significant; 20% of patients with ST segment depression and 15% of patients with inverted T waves will experience severe angina, myocardial infarction or death within 12 months of their initial presentation, compared to 10% of patients with a normal trace (Channer & Morris, 2008). It is therefore paramount that patients presenting with chest pain who have ischaemic changes on their ECG are reviewed by a cardiologist; percutaneous coronary intervention (PCI) may be indicated.

NB ST segment and T wave changes are not necessarily an indication of ischaemia; they can also be associated with left ventricular hypertrophy, digoxin toxicity and hypokalaemia.

### ST segment depression

Myocardial ischaemia typically causes ST segment depression, which can present in different ways (see Figure 11.12). In any given lead, the degree of ST segment depression is proportional to the size of the R wave, i.e. it is more prominent in leads V1–V6 (Channer & Morris, 2008).

The ECG in Figure 11.13 was recorded in a 68-year-old man complaining of chest pain during an adenosine stress test

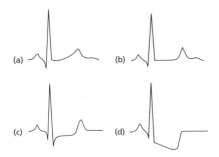

**Figure 11.12** ST changes with ischaemia showing normal wave form (a); flattening of ST segment (b), making T wave more obvious; horizontal (planar) ST segment depression (c); and downsloping ST segment depression (d). Reprinted from Morris F, *et al.*, *ABC of Clinical Electrocardiography*, 2nd edn, copyright 2008, with permission of Blackwell Publishing.

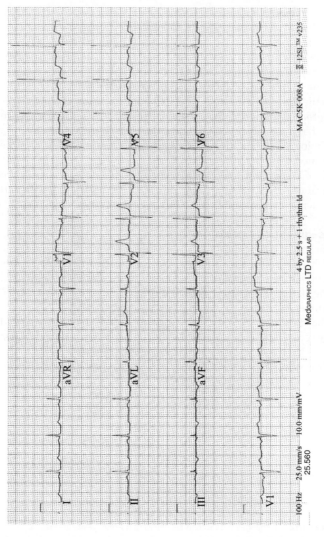

**Figure 11.13** Ischaemic changes: widespread ST segment depression.

(myoview). There are widespread ischaemic changes (ST segment depression) indicating extensive coronary disease.

### T wave changes

T wave changes associated with myocardial ischaemia can present in a variety of different ways (see Figure 11.14):

- Tall T waves – in leads V1–V3 these may be due to posterior wall myocardial ischaemia (mirror image of T wave inversion).
- Biphasic T waves – particularly seen in the anterior chest leads (see Figure 11.15).
- Inverted T waves (NB T waves can be inverted in leads III, aVR and V1 in normal individuals) (see Figure 11.16).
- Flattened T waves.

(Channer & Morris, 2008)

## ECG CHANGES ASSOCIATED WITH BUNDLE BRANCH BLOCK

### Left bundle branch block

In left bundle branch block, conduction down the left bundle branches is blocked. It is most commonly caused by ischaemic

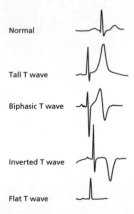

Normal

Tall T wave

Biphasic T wave

Inverted T wave

Flat T wave

**Figure 11.14** T changes associated with myocardial ischaemia. Reprinted from Morris F, *et al.*, *ABC of Clinical Electrocardiography*, 2nd edn, copyright 2008, with permission of Blackwell Publishing.

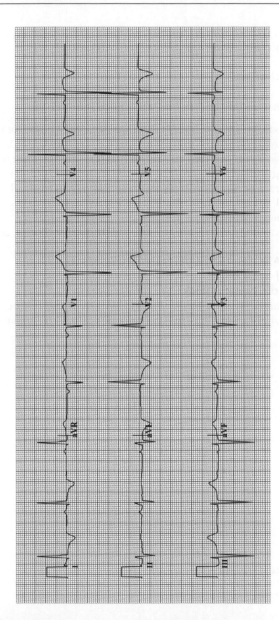

**Figure 11.15** Ischaemic changes: biphasic T waves (V2–V4) and inverted T waves (I, aVL, V5 and V6).

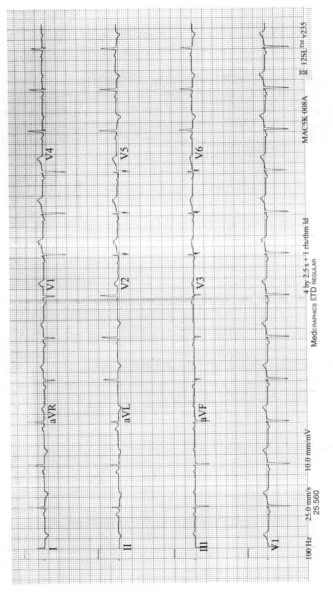

**Figure 11.16** Ischaemic changes: inverted T waves.

heart disease, hypertensive disease or dilated cardiomyopathy (Da Costa *et al.*, 2008). It is rare for left bundle branch block to be present in the absence of organic disease (Da Costa *et al.*, 2008). Diagnosis can be made by examining chest leads V1 and V6:

- Septal depolarisation occurs from right to left: small Q wave in V1 and an R wave in V6 (the direction of intraventricular depolarisation is reversed, the septal waves are lost and are replaced with R waves) (Da Costa *et al.*, 2008).
- Right ventricular depolarisation first: R wave in V1 and an S wave in V6 (often appearing as just a notch).
- Left ventricular depolarisation second: S wave in V1 and another R wave in V6.
- Delay in ventricular depolarisation leads to a wide (0.12 s/3 small squares or more) QRS complex.
- Abnormal depolarisation of the ventricles leads to secondary repolarisation changes: ST segment depression together with T wave inversion in leads with a dominant R wave; ST segment elevation and upright T waves in leads with a dominant S wave (i.e. discordance between the QRS complex and ST segment and T wave) (Da Costa *et al.*, 2008).

Left bundle branch block is best viewed in V6: the QRS complex is wide and has an M-shaped configuration. The W-shaped QRS appearance in V1 is seldom seen.

The ECG in Figure 11.17 displays left bundle branch block. The QRS width is prolonged at 0.16 s/4 small squares. The W-shaped morphology of the QRS complex in V1 and the M-shaped morphology of the QRS complex in V6 can be seen clearly.

### Right bundle branch block

In right bundle branch block, conduction down the right bundle branch is blocked. Conditions associated with right bundle branch block include ischaemic heart disease, pulmonary embolism, rheumatic heart disease and cardiomyopathy (Da Costa *et al.*, 2008). The diagnosis can be made by examining chest leads V1 and V6:

- Septal depolarisation occurs from left to right as normal: small R wave in V1 and a small Q wave in V6.

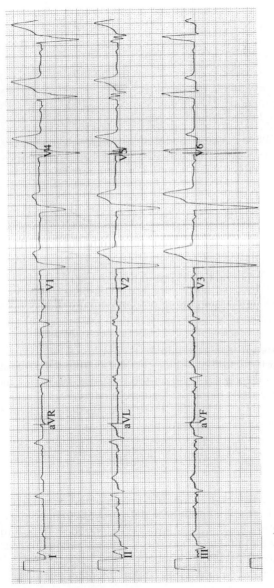

**Figure 11.17** Left bundle branch block.

- Left ventricular depolarisation first: S wave in V1 and an R wave in V6.
- Right ventricular depolarisation second: a second R wave in V1 and a deep wide S wave in V6.
- Latter part of the QRS complex is abnormal: slurred R and S waves in V1 and V6 respectively (Da Costa *et al.*, 2008).
- ST segment depression and T wave inversion in the right precordial leads (Da Costa *et al.*, 2008).

Right bundle branch block is best viewed in V1: the QRS complex is wide (0.12 s/3 small squares or more) and has a characteristic rSR pattern (see Figure 11.18).

### Left anterior fascicular block

In left anterior fascicular block (sometimes termed left anterior hemiblock), conduction down the anterior fascicle of the left bundle branch is blocked. Depolarisation of the left ventricle is via the left posterior fascicle. The cardiac axis therefore rotates in an upwards direction resulting in left axis deviation. Left anterior fascicular block is characterised by a mean frontal plane axis more leftward than 30° in the absence of inferior myocardial infarction or other cause of left axis deviation (Da Costa *et al.*, 2008).

### Left posterior fascicular block

In left posterior fascicular block (sometimes termed left posterior hemiblock), conduction down the posterior fascicle of the left bundle branch is blocked. Depolarisation of the left ventricle is via the left anterior fascicle. The cardiac axis therefore rotates in a downwards direction resulting in right axis deviation.

Left posterior fascicular block is characterised by a mean frontal plane axis of greater than 90° in the absence of another cause of right axis deviation (Da Costa *et al.*, 2008).

### Bifascicular block

In bifascicular block, there is right bundle branch block and blockage of either the left anterior or posterior fascicle (determined by the presence of left or right axis deviation respectively). Right bundle branch block together with left anterior fascicular block is the commonest type of bifascicular block (Da Costa *et al.*,

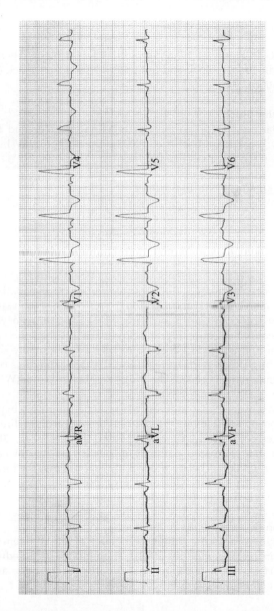

**Figure 11.18** Right bundle branch block.

2008). Bifascicular block is indicative of widespread conduction problems.

The ECG in Figure 11.19 displays bifascicular block. There is right bundle branch block and left anterior fascicular block (left axis deviation).

### Trifascicular block

Trifascicular block is when there is bifascicular block and first degree AV block (Da Costa *et al.*, 2008). Third degree AV block will ensue if the other fascicle fails as well.

### Wolff-Parkinson-White Syndrome

In 1915, Wilson described a patient with frequent attacks of rapid heart beat and an electrocardiogram which demonstrated a short P-R interval and a wide QRS complex (Wilson, 1915); in 1921, a patient with similar signs and symptoms was described by Wedd (Wedd, 1921). In 1930, Wolff and his colleagues reported a series of 11 patients who also shared similar clinical and electrocardiographic findings to those of the patients described above (Wolff *et al.*, 1930); they were young, healthy patients, usually with no underlying heart disease, who were prone to paroxysms of recurrent tachycardia and had the combination of a prolonged QRS complex and an abnormally short P-R interval. Many reports have followed, establishing this combination and referring to it as the Wolff-Parkinson-White (WPW) syndrome.

WPW syndrome is a condition where atrial impulses bypass the AV junction and activate the ventricular myocardium directly via an accessory pathway (bundle of Kent) (Fengler *et al.*, 2007). More than one accessory pathway is present in 10% of cases (Esberger *et al.*, 2008). The accessory pathway(s) allows the formation of a re-entry circuit, which can give rise to either a narrow complex or a broad complex tachycardia depending on whether the AV junction or the accessory pathway is used for antegrade conduction (Esberger *et al.*, 2008).

WPW syndrome is the commonest cause of an AV re-entrant tachycardia (Esberger *et al.*, 2008). Thought to be hereditary (Vidaillet *et al.*, 1987), its incidence is 0.1–0.3% of the population (Fengler *et al.*, 2007).

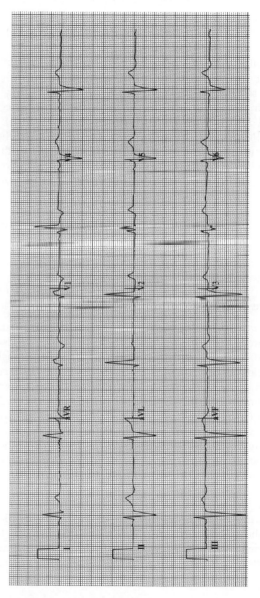

**Figure 11.19** Bifascicular block.

### Identifying ECG features

Characteristic ECG features include short PR interval (<0.12 s or 3 small squares), wide QRS complex (>0.12 s or 3 small squares) with an initial delta wave and paroxysmal tachycardia (Wolff *et al.*, 1930).

In sinus rhythm the atrial impulse is conducted rapidly down to the ventricles via the accessory pathway (it is not subjected to the normal delay as would be encountered in the AV node): hence the short PR interval. However, once the impulse reaches the ventricular myocardium, initially it is conducted (slowly) through non-specialised conduction tissue, distorting the early part of the R wave producing the characteristic delta wave (Esberger *et al.*, 2008).

WPW syndrome has traditionally been classified into two types (A and B) according to the ECG morphology in leads V1 and V2 (Esberger *et al.*, 2008; Rosenbaum *et al.*, 1945):

- *Type A*: left-sided pathway resulting in a predominant R wave (see Figure 11.20) in V1.
- *Type B*: right-sided pathway resulting in a predominant S or QS wave (see Figure 11.21) in V1.

Algorithms for the localisation of overt accessory pathways, which examine the polarity of the QRS complexes, have also been proposed (Camm & Katritsis, 1996), though none are considered very reliable (Bennett, 2006). If the accessory pathway is capable only of retrograde conduction, pre-excitation will not occur during sinus rhythm and the ECG will be normal (Esberger *et al.*, 2008).

The frequency of paroxysmal tachycardia associated with WPW syndrome increases with age (Zipes, 1992). If atrial fibrillation is present the ventricular response depends on the antegrade refractory period of the accessory pathway and may exceed 300/min resulting in ventricular fibrillation (Sharma *et al.*, 1987).

### Treatment

Patients who are symptomatic (experiencing palpitations or syncope) should be referred for electrophysiology studies (Davis, 1997). Catheter ablation, which is usually done at the same time, is highly effective in the treatment of WPW syndrome (Tishchenko *et al.*, 2008).

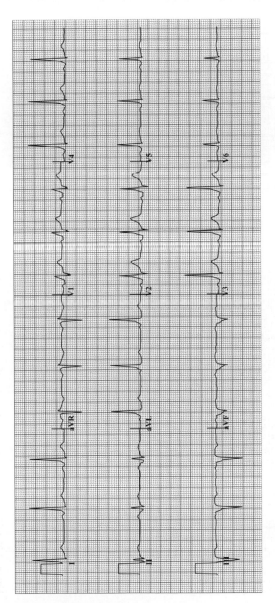

**Figure 11.20** WPW syndrome, type A (predominant R wave in V1 and V2).

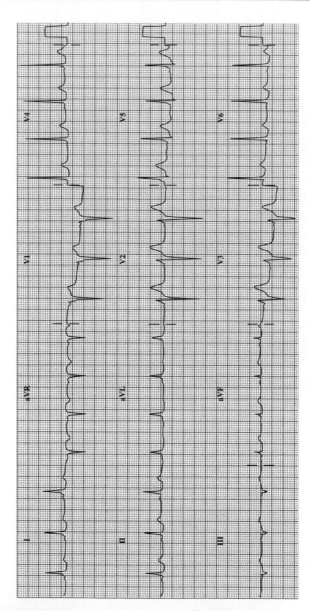

**Figure 11.21** WPW syndrome, type B (predominant S or QS wave in V1 and V2).

Drugs that block the AV node, e.g. digoxin, verapamil and adenosine, are particularly dangerous in WPW syndrome in the presence of atrial fibrillation. They decrease the refractoriness of the accessory pathways and increase the frequency of conduction, resulting in a rapid ventricular response which may lead to ventricular fibrillation (Esberger *et al.*, 2008).

## CHAPTER SUMMARY

The 12 lead ECG is an essential diagnostic tool in the management of heart disease. In particular, with the advent of thrombolytic therapy, it plays an important role in the early diagnosis of acute myocardial infarction. When interpreting a 12 lead ECG it is important to follow a systematic and logical approach.

## REFERENCES

Bennett DH (2006) *Cardiac Arrhythmias*, 6th edn. Butterworth Heinemann, Oxford.

Camm A, Katritsis D (1996) The diagnosis of tachyarrhythmias. In: Julian D, Kamm J, Fox K (eds) *Diseases of the Heart*, 2nd edn. W.B. Saunders, London.

Channer K, Morris F (2008) Myocardial ischaemia. In: Morris F, Brady W, Camm J (eds) *ABC of Clinical Electrocardiography*, 2nd edn. Blackwell Publishing, Oxford.

Colquhoun MC (1993) *A Clinical Approach to Electrocardiography*. Napp Laboratories, Cambridge.

Da Costa D, Brady W, Redhouse J (2008) Bradycardias and atrioventricular conduction block. In: Morris F, Brady W, Camm J (eds) *ABC of Clinical Electrocardiography*, 2nd edn. Blackwell Publishing, Oxford.

Davis M (1997) Catheter ablation therapy of arrhythmias. In: Thompson P (ed.) *Coronary Care Manual*. Churchill Livingstone, London.

Esberger D, Jones S, Morris F (2008) Junction tachycardias. In: Morris F, Brady W, Camm J (eds) *ABC of Clinical Electrocardiography*, 2nd edn. Blackwell Publishing, Oxford.

Fengler B, Brady W, Plautz C (2007) Wolff-Parkinson-White syndrome: ECG recognition and treatment in the ED. *American Journal of Emergency Medicine*, **25** (5), 576–583.

Hampton J (2000) *The ECG Made Easy*, 5th edn. Churchill Livingstone, London.

Houghton A, Gray D (2003) *Making Sense of the ECG*, 2nd edn. Arnold Hodder, London.

Jevon P, Ewens B (2007) *Monitoring the Critically Ill Patient*. 2nd Ed. Blackwell Publishing, Oxford.

Jevon P (2002) *Advanced Cardiac Life Support*. Butterworth Heinemann, Oxford.

Jowett NI, Thompson DR (1995) *Comprehensive Coronary Care*, 2nd edn. Scutari Press, London.

Julian D, Cowan J (1993) *Cardiology*, 6th edn. Baillière, London.

Marriott HJL (1988) *Practical Electrocardiography*, 8th edn. Williams & Wilkins, London.

Morris F, Brady W (2008) Myocardial ischaemia. In: Morris F, Brady W, Camm J, (eds) *ABC of Clinical Electrocardiography*, 2nd edn. Blackwell Publishing, Oxford.

Paul S, Hebra J (1998) *The Nurse's Guide to Cardiac Rhythm Interpretation*. W.B. Saunders, London.

Resuscitation Council UK (2006) *Advanced Life Support*, 5th edn. Resuscitation Council UK, London.

Rosenbaum F, Hecht H, Wilson F, *et al.* (1945) The potential variations of the thorax and the esophagus in anomalous atrioventricular conduction (Wolff-Parkinson-White syndromes). *American Heart Journal*, **29**, 281.

Sharma A, Yee R, Guiraudon G, Klein G (1987) Sensitivity and specificity of invasive and non-invasive testing for risk of sudden death in Wolff-Parkinson-White syndrome. *J Am Coll Cardiol*, **10**, 373.

Surawicz B, Uhley H, Borun R, *et al.* (1978) Task force 1. Standardisation of terminology and interpretation. *American Journal of Cardiology*, **41**, 130–145.

Timmis AD (1990) Early diagnosis of acute myocardial infarction. *British Medical Journal*, **301**, 941–942.

Tishchenko A, Fox D, Yee R, *et al.* (2008) When should we recommend catheter ablation for patients with the Wolff-Parkinson-White syndrome? *Current Opinion in Cardiology*; **23** (1), 32–37.

Vidaillett J, Pressley J, Henke E, *et al.* (1987) Familial occurrence of accessory atrioventricular pathways (pre-excitation syndrome). *New England Journal Medicine*, **317**, 65.

Wagner G (2000) *Practical Electrocardiography*. Williams & Wilkins, London.

Wedd A (1921) Paroxysmal tachycardia. *Archives of Internal Medicine*, **27**, 571–590.

Wilson F (1915) A case in which the vagus influenced the form of the ventricular complex of the electrocardiogram. *Archives of Internal Medicine*, **16**, 1008–1027.

Wolff L, Parkinson J, White D (1930) Bundle branch block with short PR interval in healthy young people prone to paroxysmal tachycardia. *American Heart Journal*, **5**, 685.

Zipes D (1992) Genesis of cardiac arrhythmias: electrophysiological considerations. In: Braunwald E (ed.) *Heart Disease: a Textbook of Cardiovascular Medicine*, 4th edn. W.B. Saunders, Philadelphia.

# 12 | Management of Peri-arrest Arrhythmias

## INTRODUCTION

'Peri' originates from the Greek word *peri* meaning about or around (Soanes & Stevenson, 2006). The term peri-arrest arrhythmias is used to describe cardiac arrhythmias that precede cardiac arrest or complicate the early post-resuscitation period (Colquhoun & Vincent, 2004). If untreated, they may lead to cardiac arrest or potentially avoidable deterioration in the patient (Resuscitation Council UK, 2006). Ventricular fibrillation is often triggered by a tachyarrhythmia.

The Resuscitation Council UK provides guidance for the effective and safe management of bradycardias and tachycardias (Resuscitation Council UK, 2006).

The aim of this chapter is to understand the principles of the management of peri-arrest arrhythmias.

## LEARNING OUTCOMES

At the end of the chapter the reader will be able to:

❑ Discuss the principles of the use of the peri-arrest algorithms.
❑ List the adverse clinical signs that may be associated with peri-arrest arrhythmias.
❑ Discuss the treatment options.
❑ Outline the management of bradycardia.
❑ Outline the management of tachycardia.
❑ Discuss the procedure for synchronised electrical cardioversion.
❑ Discuss the procedure for external pacing.

## PRINCIPLES OF THE USE OF THE
## PERI-ARREST ALGORITHMS

The Resuscitation Council UK's algorithms for the management of peri-arrest arrhythmias (see Figures 12.1 and 12.2) are designed for the non-specialist healthcare professional in order to provide effective and safe treatment in the emergency situation (Resuscitation Council UK, 2006). The following points regarding the use of the algorithms require emphasising:

- They are specifically designed for the peri-arrest situation and are not intended to encompass all clinical situations.
- The arrows indicate progression from one stage of treatment to the next, only if the cardiac arrhythmia persists.
- Important variables, which can influence the management, include the arrhythmia itself, the haemodynamic status of the patient, local procedures and local circumstances/facilities.
- Stated drug doses are based on average body weight and may, therefore, need adjustment in some situations.
- Anti-arrhythmic strategies can cause cardiac arrhythmias; clinical deterioration may result from the treatment itself rather than a consequence of its lack of effect.
- A high dose of a single anti-arrhythmic drug or use of different drugs can cause hypotension and myocardial depression.
- Expert help must be summoned early if simple measures are ineffective.

(Colquhoun & Vincent, 2004)

## ADVERSE CLINICAL SIGNS ASSOCIATED WITH
## PERI-ARREST ARRHYTHMIAS

The treatment for most peri-arrest arrhythmias will be dependent upon the presence or absence of certain adverse clinical signs:

- *Clinical evidence of low cardiac output*: e.g. hypotension, impaired consciousness (reduced cerebral perfusion), pallor, cold and clammy extremities.
- *Excessive tachycardia*: (typically > 150/minute) leads to a shortened diastole, which can result in a fall in cardiac output and reduced coronary blood flow (causing myocardial ischaemia).

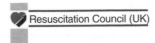

Resuscitation Council (UK)

### Adult bradycardia algorithm
(includes rates inappropriately slow for haemodynamic state)

If appropriate, give oxygen, cannulate a vein, and record a 12 lead ECG

**Adverse signs?**
- Systolic BP < 90 mmHg
- Heart rate < 40 beats min⁻¹
- Ventricular arrhythmias compromising BP
- Heart failure

**YES**      **NO**

**Atropine**
500 mcg IV

**Satisfactory response?**    **YES**

**NO**

**Risk of asystole?**
- Recent asystole
- Möbitz II AV block
- Complete heart block with broad QRS
- Ventricular pause > 3 s

**YES**

**Interim measures:**
- Atropine 500 mcg IV repeat to maximum of 3 mg
- Adrenaline 2–10 mcg min⁻¹
- Alternative drugs*
  OR
- Transcutaneous pacing

**NO**

**Observe**

**Seek expert help
Arrange transvenous pacing**

**\* Alternatives include:**
Aminophylline
Isoprenaline
Dopamine
Glucagon (if beta-blocker or calcium-channel blocker overdose)
Glycopyrrolate can be used instead of atropine

**Figure 12.1** Resuscitation Council UK Bradycardia Algorithm. Reproduced by kind permission from the Resuscitation Council UK.

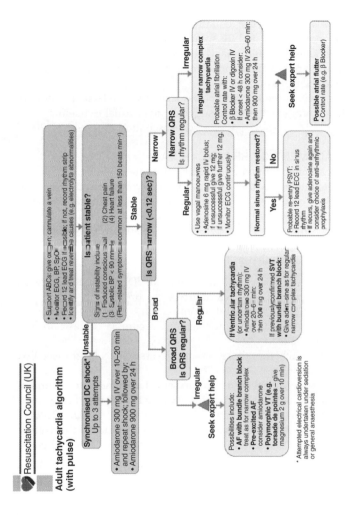

**Figure 12.2** Resuscitation Council UK Tachycardia Algorithm. Reproduced by kind permission from the Resuscitation Council UK.

- *Excessive bradycardia*: usually < 40/min, though higher rates may not be tolerated by some patients.
- *Heart failure*: – pulmonary oedema (left ventricular failure) or raised jugular venous pressure and hepatic engorgement (right ventricular failure).
- *Chest pain*: more likely to be associated with a tachyarrhythmia than a bradyarrhythmia; suggests myocardial ischaemia.

(Resuscitation Council UK, 2006)

## MANAGEMENT OF BRADYCARDIA

Bradycardia is defined as a ventricular rate < 60 per minute. An absolute rate below this level can be easily recognised. However, it is also important to identify patients with clinical evidence of critically low cardiac output in whom rates > 60 are inappropriately slow; this is termed relative bradycardia (Colquhoun & Vincent, 2004). The Resuscitation Council UK Bradycardia Algorithm is detailed in Figure 12.1).

- Assess the patient following the ABCDE approach (airway, breathing, circulation, disability, exposure).
- Administer high concentration oxygen.
- Commence ECG monitoring and secure IV access; ideally record a 12 lead ECG.
- Ascertain whether there are any adverse clinical signs (see Box 12.1).
- If adverse clinical signs are present (i.e. immediate treatment required), administer atropine 500 mcg IV; this may be repeated up to a maximum of 3 mg (Resuscitation Council UK, 2006).
- If adverse clinical signs are not present or if the administration of atropine is effective, subsequent treatment should then be

---

**Box 12.1 Bradycardia: adverse clinical signs**

Systolic blood pressure < 90 mmHg
Ventricular rate < 40/min
Ventricular arrhythmias compromising the blood pressure
Heart failure
Altered conscious level, e.g. drowsiness

---

---

**Box 12.2 Bradycardia: risk factors for asystole**

Recent asystole
Second degree AV block Mobitz II AV block
Third degree (complete) AV block, particularly if broad QRS
  complex or if heart rate < 40 minute
Ventricular standstill (pause) > 3 seconds

---

guided by the presence or absence of risk factors for asystole (see Box 12.2) (Colquhoun *et al.*, 2004).

If there has not been a satisfactory response to atropine 500 mcg IV or if there is a risk factor for asystole (see Box 12.2), the definitive treatment is transvenous pacing. While waiting for expert help, possible interim measures include

- Atropine 500 mcg IV repeated at a few minute intervals to a maximum of 3 mg (Colquhoun & Vincent, 2004).
- Transcutaneous or external pacing.
- Adrenaline infusion 2–10 mcg/min titrated to response (1 ml of 1 : 1000 adrenaline in 500 ml of 0.9% normal saline; rate 1–5 ml per min) – usually only used if transcutaneous pacing is not immediately available.
- Fist pacing.

## MANAGEMENT OF TACHYCARDIA

The Resuscitation Council UK Tachycardia Algorithm is detailed in Figure 12.2.

- Assess the patient following the ABCDE approach (airway, breathing, circulation, disability, exposure).
- Administer high concentration oxygen.
- Commence ECG monitoring and secure IV access; ideally record a 12 lead ECG.
- Ascertain whether there are any adverse clinical signs (see Box 12.3).
- If adverse clinical signs are present (i.e. immediate treatment required), perform synchronised electrical cardioversion. If this is unsuccessful, administer amiodarone 300 mg IV over

---

> **Box 12.3 Tachycardia: adverse clinical signs**
>
> Systolic blood pressure < 90 mmHg
> Heart rate > 150/min
> Heart failure
> Altered conscious level, e.g. drowsiness
> Chest pain

10–20 mins with further synchronised cardioversion if indicated, followed by 900 mg infusion over 24 hours (Resuscitation Council UK, 2006).

- If adverse clinical signs are not present, ascertain whether the QRS complex is narrow (<3 small squares or 0.12 secs) or broad, regular or irregular.

**Regular narrow complex tachycardia**

It is important to exclude sinus tachycardia which is likely to be regular, with a rate < 140/min and non-paroxysmal, i.e. it does not start and end abruptly. The treatment for sinus tachycardia is targeted at identifying and treating the cause (where appropriate).

- If there are no contraindications, try vagal manoeuvres (see Box 12.4). They are used to stimulate the vagus nerve and induce a reflex slowing of the heart (Smith, 2003). They are successful in terminating 25% of narrow complex tachycardias (Resuscitation Council UK, 2006). Caution should be exercised regarding the use of vagal manoeuvres. Profound vagal tone can induce sudden bradycardia and trigger ventricular fibrillation, particularly in the presence of digitalis toxicity or acute cardiac ischaemia (Colquhoun & Vincent, 2004).
- If vagal manoeuvres fail, and the arrhythmia is not atrial flutter, administer adenosine 6 mg IV (rapid bolus); if there is no response, administer adenosine 12 mg IV (rapid bolus). If there is no response to this, administer a further 12 mg dose IV (Resuscitation Council UK, 2006).
- If both vagal manoeuvres and adenosine are unsuccessful, seek expert help.
- If the arrhythmia is atrial flutter, seek expert help.

---

**Box 12.4 Vagal manoeuvres**

*Carotid sinus massage*: should not be used in the presence of a carotid bruit as atheromatous plaque rupture could embolise into the cerebral circulation causing a cerebral vascular accident; elderly patients are more vulnerable to plaque rupture and cerebral vascular complications (Bastuli & Orlowski, 1985; Skinner & Vincent, 1997).

*Valsalva manoeuvre*: forced expiration against a closed glottis, e.g. ask the patient to blow into a 20 ml syringe with enough force to push the plunger back (Resuscitation Council UK, 2006).

---

### Irregular narrow complex tachycardia

An irregular narrow complex tachycardia is likely to be atrial fibrillation or, rarely, atrial flutter with varying AV block; record a 12 lead ECG to assist in interpretation (Resuscitation Council UK, 2006).

If there are no adverse signs present, treatment options are:

- Drug therapy to control the ventricular rate, e.g. beta blocker, digoxin or diltiazem.
- Drug therapy to control the rhythm (chemical cardioversion).
- Synchronised electrical DC cardioversion to control the rhythm.
- Treatment to prevent complications, e.g. anti-coagulation.

(Nolan *et al.*, 2005)

Seek expert help to establish the most appropriate treatment for the patient. The longer the time the patient remains in atrial fibrillation, the greater the risk of an atrial thrombus developing; therefore:

- *Duration of atrial fibrillation > 48 hours*: as there is a risk of an atrial thrombus being present, the treatment of choice is heart rate control with anti-coagulation. Cardioversion should be deferred until the patient has been adequately coagulated (INR > 2) for at least four weeks. If early electrical or chemical cardioversion is indicated by the patient's clinical state, then the risk of stroke has to be balanced with the risk of continued atrial fibrillation. Ideally, left left atrial thrombus should be excluded with a transoesophageal echocardiogram and the patient fully coagulated with heparin.

- *Duration of atrial fibrillation < 48 hours*: if rhythm control is indicated, chemical cardioversion with amiodarone 300 mg IV over 20–60 mins, followed by 900 mg IV over 24 hours, is recommended (synchronised electrical cardioversion remains a treatment option in these patients: it is more successful than chemical cardioversion at restoring sinus rhythm).

(Nolan *et al.*, 2005)

### Regular broad complex tachycardia

A regular broad complex tachycardia is likely to be ventricular tachycardia (i.e. ventricular in origin) (Colquhoun & Vincent, 2004); if there are no adverse signs, administer amiodarone 300 mg IV over 20–60 mins, followed by an infusion of 900 mg over 24 hours (Resuscitation Council UK, 2006).

For a regular broad complex tachycardia that is considered to be supraventricular tachycardia with bundle branch block (rare), follow the protocol for regular narrow complex tachycardia described above, i.e. adenosine, etc.

### Irregular broad complex tachycardia

Seek expert help.

An irregular broad complex tachycardia could be:

- *Atrial fibrillation with bundle branch block* (most common cause): treat as for atrial fibrillation (irregular narrow complex tachycardia) (see above).
- *Atrial fibrillation in the presence of Wolf Parkinson Syndrome* (pre-excitation): greater variation in the morphology (shape) and width of the QRS complexes compared to atrial fibrillation with bundle branch block. Avoid adenosine, digoxin, verapamil and diltiazem as these drugs block the AV junction, which can cause an increase in pre-excitation; synchronised electrical cardioversion is usually the safest treatment option.
- *Polymorphic ventricular tachycardia*, e.g. torsades de points: stop all medications that can cause a prolonged QT interval, correct any electrolyte abnormalities and administer magnesium

sulphate 2 mg IV over 10 minutes; overdrive cardiac pacing is sometimes required.

(Nolan et al., 2005)

## SYNCHRONISED ELECTRICAL CARDIOVERSION

Synchronised electrical cardioversion is a reliable method of converting a tachyarrhythmia to sinus rhythm (Resuscitation Council UK, 2006). Due to the associated risks, it is generally only undertaken when pharmacological intervention has been unsuccessful, or if there are adverse signs, e.g. chest pain, hypotension, reduced level of consciousness, rapid ventricular rate and dyspnoea (Nolan *et al.*, 2005).

### Reducing transthoracic impedance

If synchronised electrical cardioversion is to be successful, sufficient electrical current needs to pass through the chest and depolarise a critical mass of myocardium. Transthoracic impedance is the resistance to the flow of current through the chest; the greater the resistance, the less the current flow. There are several factors that can influence transthoracic impedance and correct defibrillation technique is essential to minimise their effect and maximise current flow to the myocardium.

### *Electrode size*

Generally, the larger the electrodes, the lower the impedance (Deakin *et al.*, 1999), though excessively large paddles can result in decreased current flow (Deakin *et al.*, 1999). The recommended sum of the electrode areas is a minimum of $150\,cm^2$ (Association of Instrumentation, 1993). In adult defibrillation, both handheld paddle electrodes (see Figure 12.3) and self-adhesive pad electrodes (see Figure 12.4) 8–12 cm in diameter are used and function well (Resuscitation Council UK, 2006). Paediatric electrodes are associated with high impedance and, therefore, should not be used in adults when larger paddles are available.

### *Shaving the chest*

Electrode-to-skin contact can be poor if the patient has a hairy chest as air can be trapped between the electrode and the skin; this can result in increased impedance, reduced defibrillation

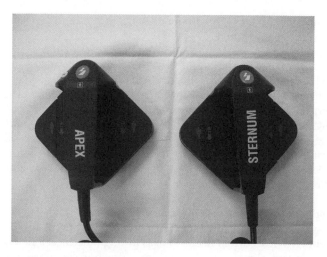

**Figure 12.3** Handheld paddle electrodes.

efficacy and arcing (sparks) causing burns to the patient's chest (Deakin & Nolan, 2005). If necessary, remove excess chest hair from the area where the electrodes are going to be placed (Resuscitation Council UK, 2006).

### Electrode paddles-skin-interface
If electrode paddles are used with no electrode-skin-interface, there will be high transthoracic impedance. Defibrillation gel pads (see Figure 12.5) should be used to reduce the impedance between the electrode paddles and the skin (they also can help prevent skin burns). Defibrillation gel is not recommended as it can be messy and any 'stray' gel can lead to arcing on the chest and reduce the efficacy of defibrillation (Deakin & Nolan, 2005).

### Large adhesive pad electrodes-skin-interface
If large adhesive pad electrodes are used, it is important to prepare the chest. Ensure the pads are in date, shave the chest if necessary (see above) and wipe the skin dry to help ensure good contact.

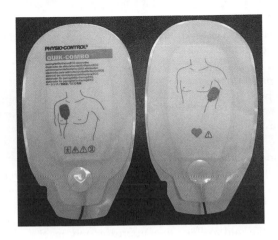

**Figure 12.4** Self-adhesive pad electrodes.

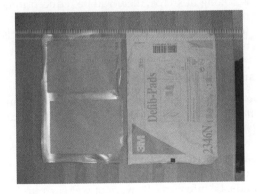

**Figure 12.5** Defibrillation gel pads.

## Electrode paddle force

If using electrode paddles, they should be pressed firmly to the chest wall. This will help to reduce impedance by improving electrical contact at the electrode-skin-interface and reducing thoracic volume. In adults, the optimal electrode paddle force is

8 kg and as this can be difficult to achieve, it is advisable for the strongest members of the cardiac arrest team to undertake this role (Deakin *et al.*, 2002).

### Phase of ventilation
Air is a poor conductor of electricity. There is reduced impedance when shocks are delivered at the end of full expiration compared to inspiration.

### Electrode position
The electrodes should be placed to maximise the current flow through the myocardium. The most commonly used electrode position is one electrode on the anterior chest, just to the right of the sternum (not over the sternum) below the right clavicle, the other in the mid-axillary line, approximately level with the V6 ECG electrode position. In women, breast tissue should be avoided as this can increase transthoracic impedance. If the apical electrode is oblong in shape, there will be reduced impedance if it is positioned longitudinally (Deakin *et al.*, 2003). The accuracy of electrode placement has been questioned and care should be taken to ensure correct placement.

### General safety issues

- Remove transdermal medication patches as they can compromise effective electrode contact and could cause arcing and burns (Wrenn, 1990).
- Avoid direct and indirect contact with the patient. All personnel should be well away from the bed and not touching the patient or anything attached to the patient/bed, e.g. IV infusion stands, IV infusions. Be wary of wet surroundings.
- Temporarily remove the oxygen delivery device at least one metre away from the patient's chest. If the patient has a self-inflating bag connected to a tracheal tube this can be left in place or removed (Resuscitation Council UK, 2006). If the patient is on a ventilator, leave the ventilator tubing connected (Deakin & Nolan, 2005).
- Shout 'stand clear' and check all personnel are safely clear prior to defibrillation. No person should be touching the

patient or anything in contact with the patient, e.g. bed, drip stand.

- Check the ECG monitor immediately prior to defibrillation; sometimes the ECG can revert to a sinus rhythm.
- Place the electrode paddles or pads 12 to 15 cm away from an implanted pacing unit (Resuscitation Council UK, 2006) (most pacemaker units are below the left clavicle, therefore the standard defibrillation can be adopted, if below the right clavicle the anterior-posterior paddle position may be necessary).
- Minimise the risk of sparks during defibrillation: in theory, there is a decreased risk of this when using self-adhesive pad electrodes compared to paddle electrodes (Deakin & Nolan, 2005).

### Safety issues associated with electrode paddles

- Ensure defibrillation gel pads are applied to the patient's bare chest to minimise the risk of skin burns (and improve conduction).
- Apply adequate pressure to the paddles (8 kg) to help minimise the risk of arcing (Deakin et al., 2002).
- Charge the defibrillator with the electrode paddles on the patient's chest. This will avoid moving charged paddles between their storage site and the patient's chest.
- If indicated, ask a colleague to increase the energy level on the defibrillator (if alone, return one electrode paddle to the defibrillator and use the free hand to increase the energy level).

### Electrode pads or paddles

Self-adhesive pad electrodes are safe, effective and preferable to paddle electrodes (Stults et al., 1987). They enable the operator to defibrillate the patient 'hands-free' at a distance (electrode paddles require the operator to lean over the patient – hazardous).

### Synchronisation with the R wave

The shock must be delivered with the R wave and not the T wave (Deakin & Nolan, 2005), as delivery of the shock during the refractory period of the cardiac cycle (T wave) could induce ventricular fibrillation (Lown, 1967). The defibrillator must therefore be synchronised with the patient's electrocardiogram.

In pulseless ventricular tachycardia, synchronisation is not required. The defibrillator will not be able to synchronise in ventricular fibrillation as there are no recognisable R waves (Resuscitation Council UK, 2006).

## Monophasic and biphasic waveforms

For cardioversion of a broad complex tachycardia and atrial fibrillation, an initial 120–150 joules (J) biphasic (200 J monophasic) shock is recommended. For cardioversion of a regular narrow complex tachycardia or atrial flutter, lower energy levels are usually successful. An initial shock at 70–120 J biphasic or 100 J monophasic is recommended (Resuscitation Council UK, 2005).

## Atrial fibrillation and the risk of cerebral embolism

Due to the risk of a cerebral or peripheral embolism arising from stasis of blood and subsequent thrombosis in the left atrium, a patient who has had atrial fibrillation for more than 48 hours should normally not receive synchronised electrical cardioversion (see pages 227–8) (Resuscitation Council UK, 2006).

## Procedure of synchronised electrical cardioversion (electrode paddles)

(1) Record a 12 lead ECG, unless the patient is severely compromised and doing so will delay the procedure.

(2) Explain the procedure to the patient. Written informed consent should be obtained if possible. If the patient is not unconscious, he must be anaesthetised or sedated for the procedure (Nolan *et al.*, 2005).

(3) If necessary, shave the patient's chest (see above) as this can reduce transthoracic impedance (Sado *et al.*, 2004).

(4) Ensure the resuscitation equipment is immediately available.

(5) Establish ECG monitoring using the defibrillator that will be used for cardioversion.

(6) Select an ECG monitoring lead that will provide a clear ECG trace, e.g. lead II.

(7) Press the 'synch' button on the defibrillator (see Figure 12.6). The defibrillator should identify each R wave.

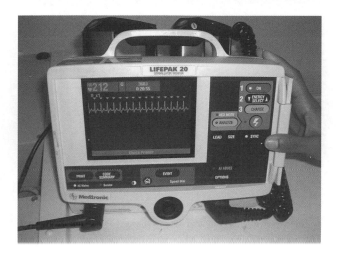

**Figure 12.6** Electrical cardioversion: activating the synchronised button.

(8) Check the ECG trace to ensure that only the R waves are being synchronised (see Figure 12.7), i.e. a 'synchronised' dot or arrow should appear on each R wave and nowhere else on the PQRST cycle, e.g. on tall T waves.

(9) Apply defibrillation gel pads to the patient's chest, one just to the right of the sternum, below the right clavicle, and the other in the mid-axillary line, approximately level with the V6 ECG electrode or female breast (Deakin & Nolan, 2005).

(10) Select the appropriate energy level on the defibrillator (see above for recommended levels).

(11) Position the defibrillator paddles firmly on the defibrillation pads.

(12) Charge the defibrillator and shout 'stand clear'.

(13) Check all personnel are safely clear prior to defibrillation (see Figure 12.8). No person should be touching the patient or anything in contact with the patient, e.g. bed, drip stand.

(14) Check the ECG monitor to ensure that the patient is still in the tachyarrhythmia that requires cardioversion, that the synchronised button remains activated and that it is still synchronising with the R waves.

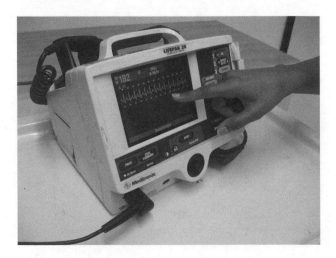

**Figure 12.7** Electrical cardioversion: check the ECG trace to ensure that only the R waves are being synchronised.

(15) Press both discharge buttons simultaneously to discharge the shock. There is usually a slight delay between pressing the shock buttons and shock discharge.

(16) Re-assess the ECG trace. The 'synch' button will usually need to be reactivated if further cardioversion is required (on some defibrillators it is necessary to actually switch off the 'synch' button if further cardioversion is not indicated). Stepwise increases in energy will be required if cardioversion needs to be repeated (Deakin & Nolan, 2005). Amiodarone is indicated if three attempts at cardioversion have been unsuccessful (Nolan *et al.*, 2005).

(17) After successful cardioversion, record a 12 lead ECG.

(18) Monitor the patient's vital signs until they have fully recovered from the anaesthetic or sedative.

### Procedure for synchronised electrical cardioversion (large adhesive pad electrodes)

If large adhesive pad electrodes are to be used, attach the cable from the defibrillator to the pads (hands-free system) and follow

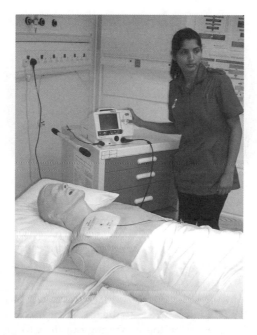

**Figure 12.8** Electrical cardioversion: check all personnel are safely clear prior to delivering the shock.

the above procedure; defibrillation gel pads and paddles are not required.

### Implantable cardioverter defibrillator

The implantable cardioverter defibrillator (ICD) (see Figure 12.9) can be used in patients with recurrent life-threatening ventricular arrhythmias who have not responded to conventional treatment. Its use is associated with improved chances of survival (Resuscitation Council UK, 2006).

The ICD is positioned in a similar position to permanent pacemakers and can provide over-ride pacing, low-energy synchronised cardioversion, high-energy defibrillation and pacing for bradycardia (Causer & Connelly, 1998).

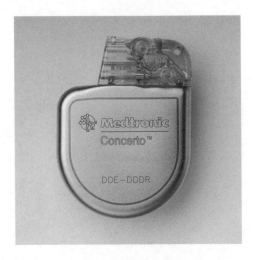

**Figure 12.9** Implantable cardioverter defibrillator (ICD).

If a patient with an ICD has a cardiac arrest, standard CPR can be carried out without any risks to the team. If the ICD discharges it will not be detected by those carrying out the CPR. If external defibrillation is indicated, the paddles should be placed 12–15 cm away from the unit (Resuscitation Council UK, 2006).

## PRINCIPLES OF EXTERNAL PACING

Cardiac pacing is the delivery of a small electrical current to the heart to stimulate myocardial contraction. External (transcutaneous or percussion) pacing can be established quickly and easily during CPR. It buys time for the spontaneous recovery of the conduction system or for more definitive treatment to be established, e.g. transvenous pacing.

### Indications

- *Profound bradycardia*: e.g. sometimes found in complete heart block, that has not responded to pharmacological treatment, e.g. atropine. NB If the intrinsic QRS complexes are not associated with a pulse (pulseless electrical activity or PEA), attempts at pacing will be futile.

- *Ventricular standstill*: P waves (atrial contraction) only on the ECG.

NB Although pacing is not indicated in asystole, always check the ECG carefully for the presence of P waves (ventricular standstill) as this may respond to pacing (Nolan *et al.*, 2005).

### Advantages of trancutaneous pacing

- Can be quickly established.
- Easy to undertake, requiring minimal training.
- Risks associated with central venous cannulation are avoided.
- Can be undertaken by nurses.

(Resuscitation Council UK, 2006)

### Procedure for transcutaneous pacing

- If appropriate, explain the procedure to the patient.
- Ideally, first remove excess chest hair from the pacing electrode sites by clipping close to the patient's skin using a pair of scissors (shaving the skin is not recommended as any nicks in the skin can lead to burns and pain during pacing) (Resuscitation Council UK, 2006).
- Attach the pacing electrodes following the manufacturer's instructions.
- Pacing-only electrodes: attach the anterior electrode on the left anterior chest, midway between the xiphoid process and the left nipple (V2–V3 ECG electrode position) and attach the posterior electrode below the left scapula, lateral to the spine and at the same level as the anterior electrode – this anterior/posterior configuration will ensure that the position of the electrodes does not interfere with defibrillation (Resuscitation Council UK, 2006). ECG monitoring will usually need to be established if an older pacing system is used (Resuscitation Council UK, 2006).
- Multifunctional electrodes (pacing and defibrillation): place the anterior electrode below the right clavicle and the lateral electrode in the mid-axillary line lateral to the left nipple (V6 ECG electrode position) – this anterior-lateral position is convenient during CPR as chest compressions do not have to be interrupted (Resuscitation Council UK, 2006).

- Check that the pacing electrodes and connecting cables are applied following the manufacturer's recommendations: if they are reversed pacing may either be ineffective or high capture thresholds may be required (Resuscitation Council UK, 2006).
- Adjust the ECG gain (size) accordingly. This will help ensure that the intrinsic QRS complexes are sensed.
- Select on-demand mode on the pacing unit on the defibrillator. This results in pacing only in the absence of intrinsic electrical activity.
- Select an appropriate rate for external pacing, usually 60–90 per minute.
- Set the pacing current at the lowest level, turn on the pacemaker unit and while observing both the patient and the ECG, gradually increase the current until electrical capture occurs (QRS complexes following the pacing spike). Electrical capture usually occurs when the current delivered is in the range of 50–100 mA (Resuscitation Council UK, 2006).
- Check the patient's pulse. If he has a palpable pulse (mechanical capture), request expert help and prepare for transvenous pacing. If there is no pulse, start CPR. If there is good electrical capture, but no mechanical capture, this is indicative of a non-viable myocardium (Resuscitation Council UK, 2006). NB there is no electrical hazard if in contact with the patient during pacing (Resuscitation Council UK, 2006).

**Cautions**

- If the patient is conscious, analgesia and sedation will usually be required.
- If pacing-only electrodes have been applied and defibrillation is subsequently indicated, position the defibrillation paddles least 2–3 cm away from the pacing electrodes to avoid arching.
- Turn off pacemaker unit during CPR to prevent inappropriate stimulation of the patient (Resuscitation Council UK, 2006).

**Percussion pacing**

Percussion pacing can result in a cardiac output with minimal trauma to the patient. It is likely to be successful when there is ventricular standstill (P waves, but no QRS complexes).

It involves the delivery of gentle blows (from a height of only a few inches above the chest) over the precordium lateral to the lower left sternal edge (Resuscitation Council UK, 2006). Trial and error will determine the optimum place for percussion. Assess the patient's pulse to ensure the effectiveness of the percussion pacing.

## CHAPTER SUMMARY

A successful strategy, to reduce the mortality and morbidity of cardiac arrest, must include the effective management of peri-arrest arrhythmias. In this chapter the Resuscitation Council UK guidelines for the management of bradycardias and tachycardias have been outlined. Always seek expert help when necessary.

## REFERENCES

Association of Instrumentation (1993) *American National Standard: Automatic External Defibrillators and Remote Controlled Defibrillators (DF39).* Association of Instrumentation, Virginia.

Bastuli J, Orlowski J (1985) Stroke as a complication of carotid sinus massage. *Critical Care Medicine*, **13**, 869.

Causer J, Connelly D. (1998) Implantable defibrillators for life-threatening ventricular arrhythmias. *British Medical Journal*, **317**, 762–763.

Colquhoun M, Vincent R (2004) Management of peri-arrest arrhythmias in Colquhoun M, Handley A, Evans T (eds) *ABC of Resuscitation*, 5th edn. Blackwell Publishing, Oxford.

Deakin C, Nolan J (2005) European Resuscitation Council guidelines for resuscitation 2005: Section 3. Electrical therapies: automated external defibrillators, defibrillation, cardioversion and pacing. *Resuscitation*, **675S**, S25–S37.

Deakin C, McLaren R, Petley G, *et al.* (1999) A comparison of transthoracic impedance using standard defibrillation paddles and self-adhesive defibrillation pads. *Resuscitation*, **39**, 43–46.

Deakin C, Sado D, Petley G, Clewlow F (2002) Determining the optimal paddle force for external defibrillation. *Am J Cardiol*, **90**, 812–813.

Deakin C, Sado D, Petley G, Clewlow F (2003) Is the orientation of the apical defibrillation paddle of importance during manual external defibrillation? *Resuscitation*, **56**, 15–18.

Lown B (1967) Electrical reversion of cardiac arrhythmias. *British Heart Journal*, **29**, 469–489.

Nolan J, Deakin C, Soar J, *et al.* (2005) European Resuscitation Council Guidelines for Resuscitation 2005: Section 4. Adult advanced life support. *Resuscitation*, **675S**, S39–S86.

Resuscitation Council UK (2005) *Resuscitation Guidelines 2005*. Resuscitation Council UK, London.

Resuscitation Council UK (2006) *Advanced Life Support*, 5th edn. Resuscitation Council UK, London.

Sado D, Deakin C, Petley G, Clewlow F (2004) Comparison of the effects of removal of chest hair with not doing so before external defibrillation on transthoracic impedance. *Am J Cardiol*, **93**, 98–100.

Smith G (2003) *ALERT Acute Life-Threatening Events Recognition and Treatment*, 2nd edn. University of Portsmouth, Portsmouth.

Soanes C, Stevenson A (2006) *Oxford Dictionary of English*. Oxford University Press, Oxford.

Skinner D, Vincent R (1997) *Cardiopulmonary Resuscitation*. Oxford University Press, Oxford.

Stults K, Brown D, Cooley F, Kerber R (1987) Self-adhesive monitor/defibrillation pads improve prehospital defibrillation success. *Ann Emerg Med*, **16**, 872–877.

Wrenn K (1990) The hazards of defibrillation through nitroglycerin patches. *Am Emerg Med*, **19**, 1327–1328.

# Record Keeping

# 13

## INTRODUCTION

Good record keeping is a fundamental part of the nursing (NMC, 2005; 2008). An accurate written record detailing relevant information concerning ECG monitoring and the recording of 12 lead ECGs is important, not only because it forms an integral part of the nursing management of the patient, but also because it can help to protect the nurse if defence of her action is required. The Clinical Negligence Scheme for Trusts (CNST) also requires its members to maintain high standards of record keeping (Dimond, 2005).

The aim of this chapter is to understand the principles of good record keeping

## LEARNING OUTCOMES

At the end of the chapter the reader will be able to:

❑ Discuss the importance of good record keeping.
❑ List the common deficiencies of record keeping.
❑ Outline the principles of good record keeping.
❑ State what should be documented on a 12 lead ECG and on an ECG rhythm strip.
❑ Outline the importance of auditing records.
❑ Discuss the legal issues associated with record keeping.

## IMPORTANCE OF GOOD RECORD KEEPING

*Record keeping is an integral part of nursing, midwifery and health visiting practice. It is a tool of professional practice and one that should help the care process. It is not separate from this process and it is not an optional extra to be fitted in if circumstances allow.*

(NMC, 2005).

Good record keeping will help to protect the welfare of both the patient and practitioner by promoting:

- High standards of clinical care.
- Continuity of care.
- Better communication and dissemination of information between members of the inter-professional healthcare team.
- The ability to detect problems, such as changes in the patient's condition at an early stage.
- An accurate account of treatment and care planning and delivery.

The quality of record keeping is also a reflection on the standard of nursing practice: good record keeping is an indication that the practitioner is professional and skilled, while poor record keeping often highlights wider problems with the individual's practice (NMC, 2005).

## COMMON DEFICIENCIES IN RECORD KEEPING

Nearly every report published by the Health Service Commissioner (Health Service Ombudsman) following a complaint identifies examples of poor record keeping that has either hampered the care the patient has received or has made it difficult for healthcare professionals to defend their practice (Dimond, 2005).

Common deficiencies in record keeping encountered include:

- Absence of clarity.
- Failure to record action taken when a problem has been identified.
- Missing information.
- Spelling mistakes.
- Inaccurate records.

(Dimond, 2005)

## PRINCIPLES OF GOOD RECORD KEEPING

There are a number of factors that underpin good record keeping. The patient's records should:

- Be factual, consistent and accurate.
- Be updated as soon as possible after any recordable event.

- Provide current information on the care and condition of the patient.
- Be documented clearly and in such a way that the text cannot be erased.
- Be consecutive and accurately dated, timed and signed (including a printed signature).
- Have any alterations and additions dated, timed and signed; all original entries should be clearly legible.
- Not include abbreviations, jargon, meaningless phrases, irrelevant speculation and offensive subjective statements.
- Still be legible if photocopied.
- Identify any problems identified and most importantly the action taken to rectify them.

**Best practice – record keeping**

Records must be:

- Factual.
- Legible.
- Clear.
- Concise.
- Accurate.
- Signed.
- Timed.
- Dated.

(Drew *et al.*, 2000)

## WHAT SHOULD BE DOCUMENTED ON A 12 LEAD ECG AND ON AN ECG RHYTHM STRIP

It is important to record all the necessary information documented on the 12 lead ECG. In most situations this will be done electronically. However, the nurse should check that the following have been recorded:

- Patient's personal details, e.g. name, unit number, date of birth.
- Date and time of recording, together with any relevant information, e.g. if the patient was complaining of chest pain during the recording, post-thrombolysis.
- The leads (limb and chest) are correctly labelled.

- If there are changes to the standard recording, e.g. right-sided chest leads, paper speed of 50 mm/s.
- The ECG is stored in the appropriate place in the patient's notes, in chronological order with other ECGs.

ECG rhythm strips will also need to be correctly labelled and filed in the patient's notes in a chronological order. It is also important to ensure that an accurate record is made in the patient's notes. In particular, it is important to include interventions and any response to the interventions.

## IMPORTANCE OF AUDITING RECORDS
Audit can play an important role in ensuring quality of health care. In particular, it can help to improve the process of record keeping. By auditing records the standard can be evaluated and any areas for improvement and staff development identified. Audit tools should be developed at a local level to monitor the standards of record keeping.

Audit should primarily be aimed at serving the interests of the patient rather than the organisation (NMC, 2005). A system of peer review may also be of value. Whatever audit system is used, the confidentiality of patients' information applies to audit just as it does to record keeping.

## LEGAL ISSUES ASSOCIATED WITH RECORD KEEPING
The patient's records are occasionally required as evidence before a court of law, by the Health Service Commissioner or in order to investigate a complaint at a local level. Sometimes, they may be requested by the NMC's Fitness to Practice committees when investigating complaints related to misconduct. Care plans, diaries and anything that makes reference to the patient's care may be required as evidence (NMC, 2005).

What constitutes a legal document is often a cause for concern. Any document requested by the court becomes a legal document (Dimond, 1994), e.g. 12 lead ECG recording, nursing records, medical records, X-rays, laboratory reports, observation charts; in fact, any document which may be relevant to the case.

If any of the documents are missing, the writer of the records may be cross-examined as to the circumstances of their disappearance (Dimond, 1994). 'Medical records are not proof of the truth of the facts stated in them but the maker of the records may be called to give evidence as to the truth as to what is contained in them' (Dimond, 1994).

The approach to record keeping which courts of law adopt tends to be that if it is not recorded, it has not been undertaken (NMC, 2005). Professional judgement is required when deciding what is relevant and what needs to be recorded, particularly if the patient's clinical condition is apparently unchanging and no record has been made of the care that has been delivered.

A registered nurse has both a professional and a legal duty of care. Consequently, when keeping records it is important to be able to demonstrate that:

- A comprehensive nursing assessment of the patient has been undertaken including care that has been planned and provided.
- Relevant information is included together with any measures that have been taken in response to changes in the patient's condition.
- The duty of care owed to the patient has been honoured and that no acts or omissions have compromised the patient's safety.
- Arrangements have been made for ongoing care of the patient.

The registered nurse is also accountable for any delegation of record keeping to members of the multi-professional team who are not registered practitioners. For example, if record keeping is delegated to a pre-registration student nurse or a healthcare assistant, competence to perform the task must be ensured and adequate supervision provided. All such entries must be countersigned.

The Access to Health Records Act 1990 gives patients the right of access to their manually maintained health records which were made after 1 November 1991. The Data Protection Act 1998 gives patients the right to access their computer-held records. The Freedom of Information Act 2000 grants the rights to anyone to all information that is not covered by the Data Protection Act 1998 (NMC, 2005).

Sometimes, it is necessary to withhold information, if it could affect the physical or mental well-being of the patient or if it would breach another patient's confidentiality (NMC, 2005). If the decision to withhold information is made, justification for doing so must be clearly recorded in the patient's notes.

## CONCLUSION

When undertaking ECG monitoring or recording a 12 lead ECG, it is important to ensure good record keeping. Good record keeping is both the product of good teamwork and an important tool in promoting high quality health care.

## REFERENCES

Dimond B (1994) *Legal Aspects in Midwifery*. Books for Midwives. Midwifery Press, Cheshire.

Dimond B (2005) Exploring common deficiencies that occur in record keeping. *British Journal of Nursing*, **14** (10), 568–570.

Drew D, Jevon P, Raby M (2000) *Resuscitation of the Newborn*. Butterworth Heinemann, Oxford.

NMC (2005) *Guidelines for Records and Record Keeping*. NMC, London.

NMC (2008) *The Code: Standards of Conduct, Performance and Ethics for Nurses and Midwives*. NMC, London.

# Appendix

## 12 LEAD ECGS FOR INTERPRETATION

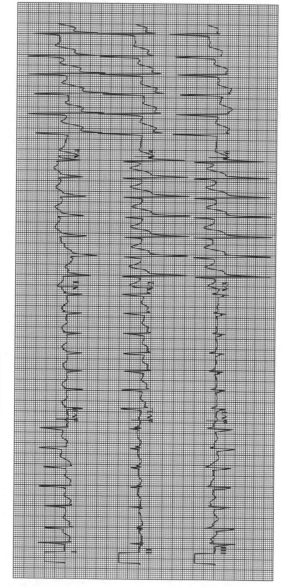

ECG 1 displays junctional tachycardia with associated widespread ST depression suggestive of myocardial ischaemia. This patient was complaining of chest pain and palpitations. Following the administration of adenosine, the ECG reverted to sinus rhythm (see Figure 11.16). However, ST depression is still evident in the lateral leads (V4, V5 and V6). This patient required further investigations for the presence of ischaemic heart disease and left ventricular hypertrophy.

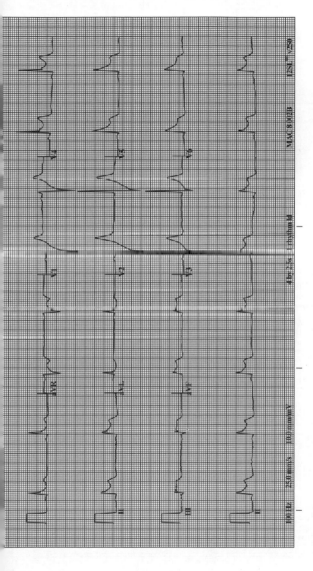

**ECG 2** displays the characteristic ECG changes associated with inferolateral myocardial infarction with probable posterior involvement as well. There is ST elevation in leads II, III, aVF, V4, V5 and V6 (inferolateral). Tall R waves and reciprocal changes in V2 and V3 are suggestive of posterior involvement as well. There is also sinus bradycardia which commonly accompanies inferior myocardial infarction. Following the administration of diamorphine the ST elevation on the cardiac monitor settled. A repeat ECG (see Figure 11.18) was recorded, which showed that the ST elevation had resolved. The diagnosis is probably Prinzmetal angina caused by transient coronary artery spasm.

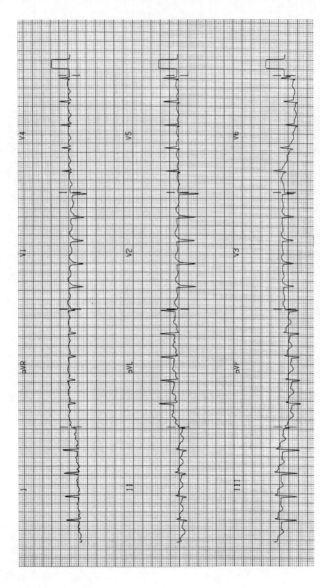

**ECG 3** displays atrial tachycardia with 2:1 AV block. The P waves are clearly visible in leads I, II and aVL. There are also pathological Q waves in leads II, III and aVF suggestive of an old inferior myocardial infarction.

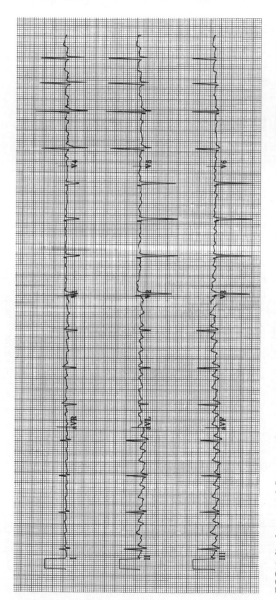

**ECG 4** displays atrial flutter with 3:1 AV block. The flutter waves are easily recognised in the inferior leads (II, III and aVF).

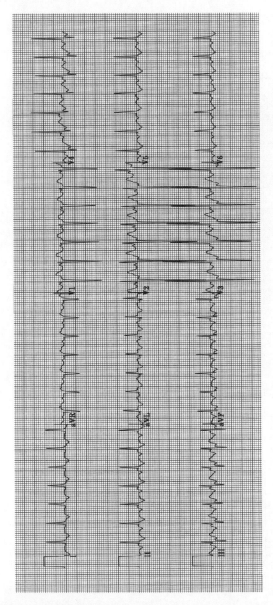

ECG 5 displays atrial flutter with 2:1 AV block resulting in a rapid ventricular response (approximately 160/min). The flutter waves can be identified in lead aVR. The rate of the flutter waves is approximately 300/min, a distinguishable feature of atrial flutter. The atrial rate is too fast for atrial tachycardia.

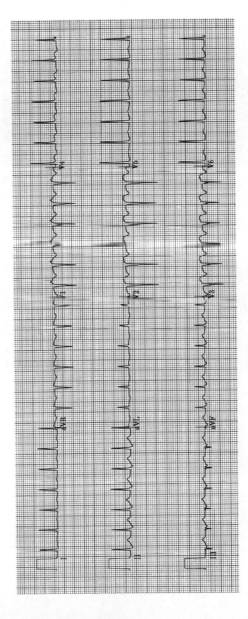

**ECG 6** displays junctional tachycardia. The narrow QRS complex is indicative of a supraventricular arrhythmia. Retrograde conducted P waves, a characteristic feature of a junctional arrhythmia, can clearly be identified in leads V1–V3. Additional anterior Q waves with minor ST elevation is also present.

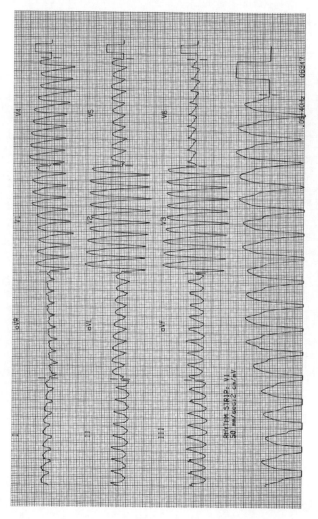

ECG 7 displays ventricular tachycardia rate approximately 220/min. The QRS complexes are wide (>0.12s/3 small squares) and there is AV dissociation (P waves are clearly visible in the rhythm strip (calibration changed to help their identification). In addition, there is right axis deviation (if the tachycardia was supraventricular in origin with left bundle branch block, then left axis deviation would be expected).

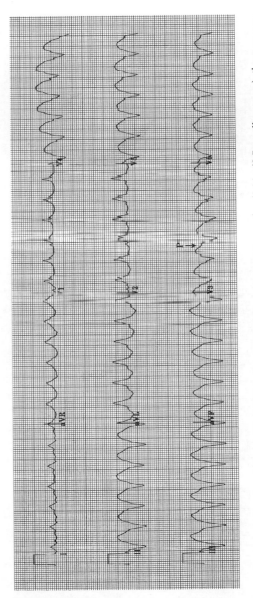

**ECG 8** displays ventricular tachycardia. This is indicated by a wide QRS complex (0.14 s/3.5 small squares), the presence of AV dissociation and the extreme left axis deviation with a positive aVR.

257

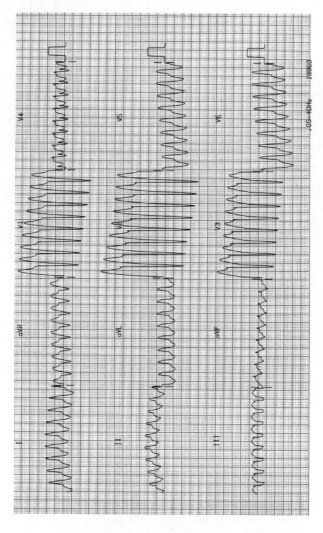

**ECG 9** displays a broad complex tachycardia caused by a junctional tachycardia with aberration. There is borderline left bundle branch block pattern with a normal axis. No identifiable P waves.

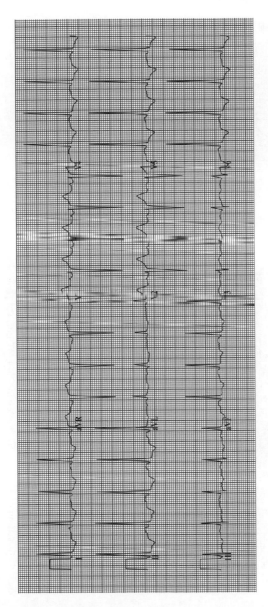

**ECG 10** displays left ventricular hypertrophy (LVH). Chest leads facing the left ventricle (V5 and V6) display abnormally tall R waves (>25 mm) and inverted T waves. The chest lead facing the right ventricle (V1) displays an abnormally deep S wave (25 mm). LVH is often associated with lateral ST depression and T wave inversion, referred to as a strain pattern.

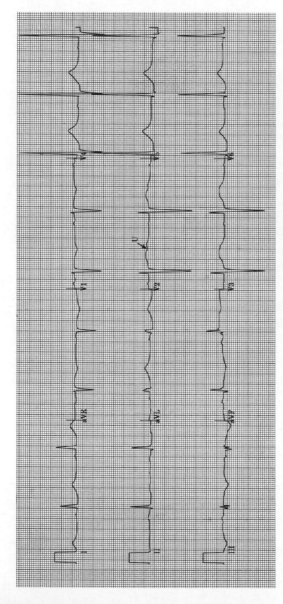

ECG 11 displays ECG changes associated with hypokalaemia. On close inspection, U waves can be identified in V2 and V3, which is characteristic of hypokalaemia. This patient's serum potassium was 2.6 mmol/litre. Additional features include flattening of T waves, ST depression and QT interval prolongation.

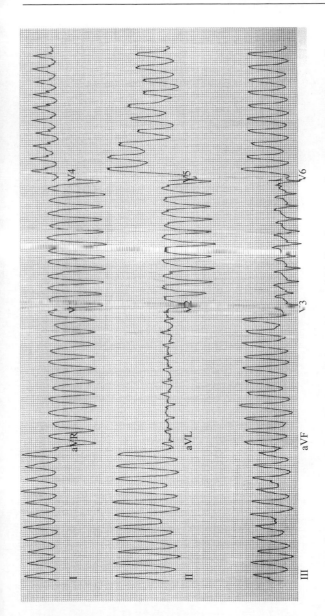

**ECG 12** displays ventricular tachycardia. Recorded in a 44-year-old lady who was undergoing an exercise test, it was self-terminating and no treatment was required. She had originally presented with a history of dizzy spells while under-taking housework. An echocardiogram and angiography were normal. Diagnosis was exercise-induced ventricular tachy-cardia. She was started on a beta blocker.

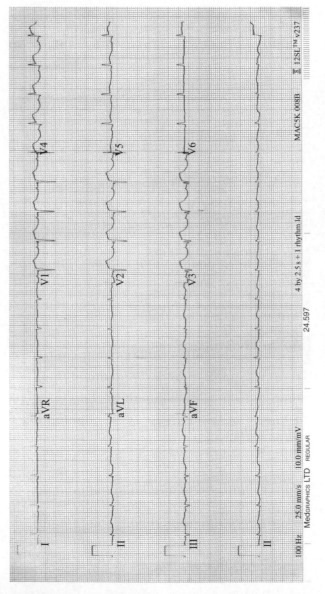

**ECG 13** displays anteroseptal myocardial infarction. It was recorded in a 72-year-old man on a ventilator on ITU four days post infarction and cardiac arrest (ventricular tachycardia) while walking around town. He received thrombolysis in A & E. The ECG shows persistent ST elevation. It is an abnormally low voltage ECG, which may accompany a very large myocardial infarction. Other causes include obesity, COPD and pericardial or pleural effusion.

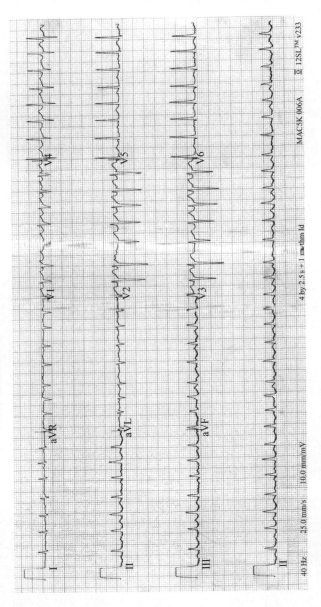

**ECG 14** displays atrial fibrillation with a fast ventricular response (190 per minute).

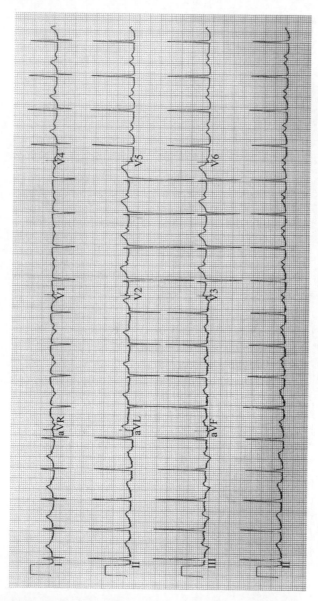

**ECG 15** displays marked first degree AV block (PR interval 250 ms). It was recorded in a 24-year-old lady admitted with a pyrexia and non-blanching rash. She was subsequently diagnosed with aortic valve endocarditis. She had developed an aortic root abscess which encroached on the bundle of His, causing first degree AV block.

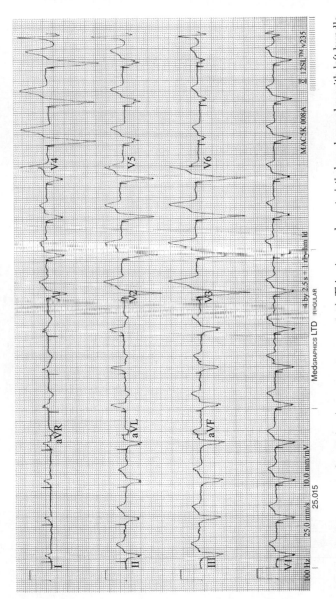

**ECG 16** displays ventricular pacing (permanent pacemaker). This gives a characteristic broad complex with left bundle branch morphology which follows a pacing spike.

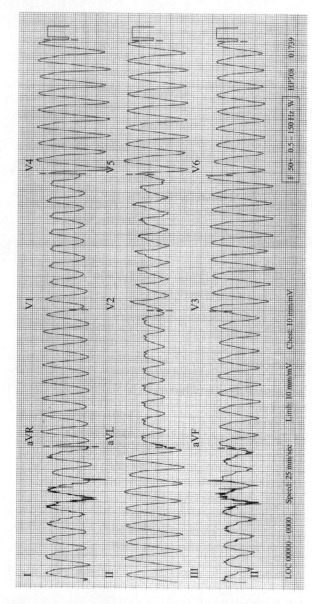

**ECG 17** displays ventricular tachycardia. The ECG was recorded in an 85- year-old man who had been admitted to the acute stroke unit. He was breathless and pale.

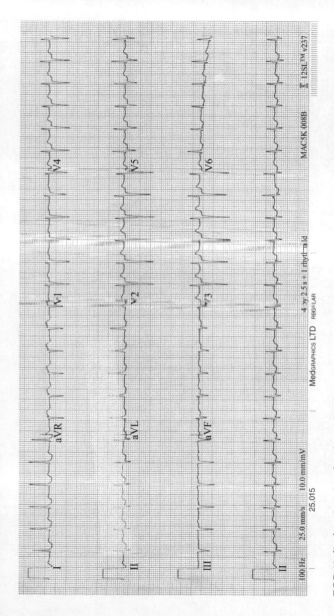

**ECG 18** displays junctional tachycardia. It was recorded in a 77-year-old lady who was receiving IV chemotherapy. She was complaining of palpitations and chest tightness. There are widespread ischaemic changes (ST depression) on the ECG (adverse sign) and the cardiologist was asked to review the patient.

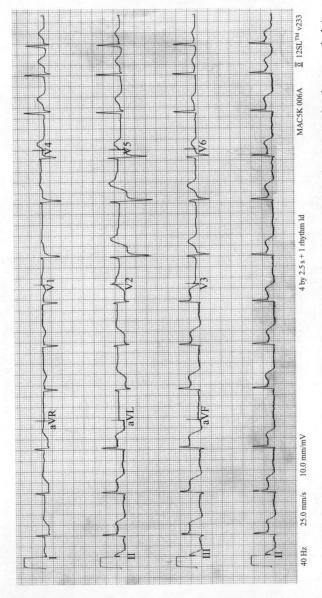

**ECG 19** displays acute inferior/posterior myocardial infarction. The ventricular rhythm is irregular due to underlying atrial fibrillation.

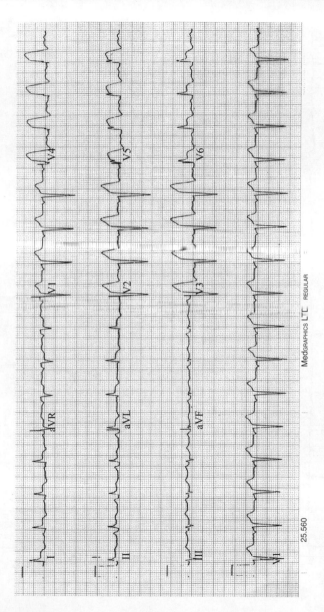

**ECG 20** displays extensive acute anterior lateral ST elevation myocardial infarction.

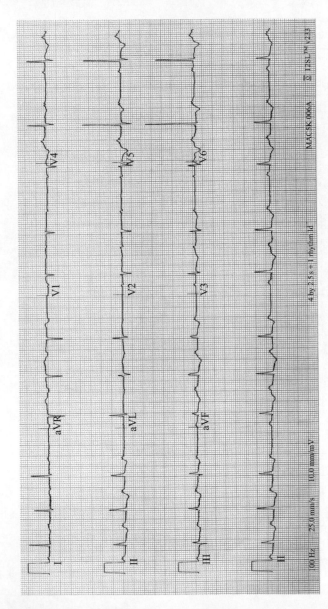

ECG 21 displays inferolateral ischaemic changes. The rhythm is second degree AV block Mobitz type 1 (Wenckeback).

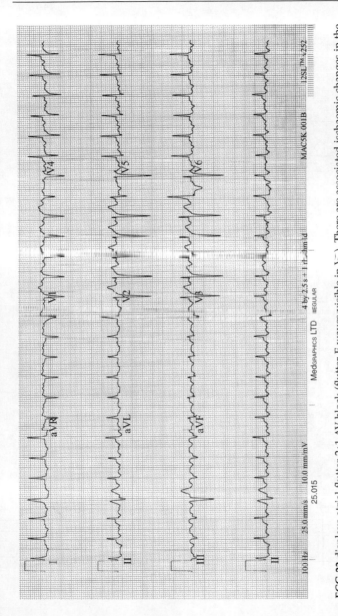

**ECG 22** displays atrial flutter 2:1 AV block (flutter F waves visible in V⁻). There are associated ischaemic changes in the anterolateral leads.

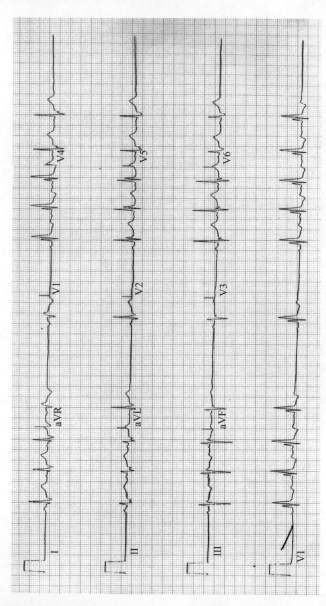

ECG 23 displays profound sinus arrhythmia. It was recorded in a patient who was hyperventilating.

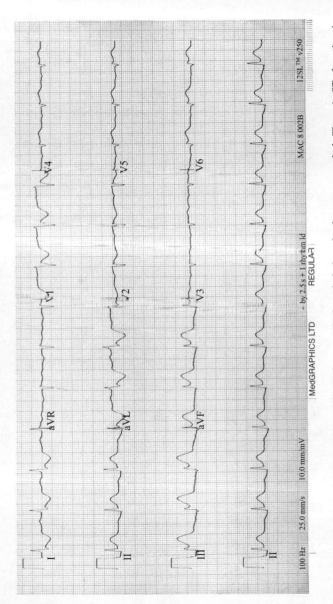

**ECG 24** displays acute inferior myocardial infarction. Right-sided chest leads were recorded. There is ST elevation in RV4–RV6 indicating right ventricular infarction.

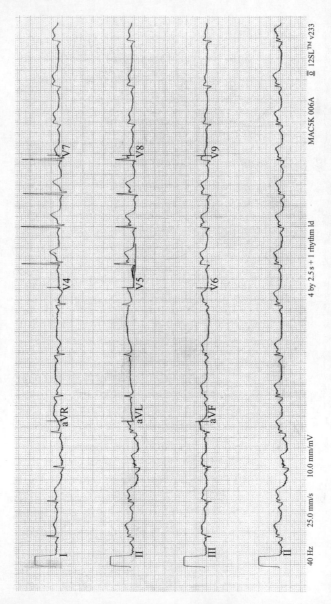

**ECG 25** displays extensive acute inferolateral and posterior myocardial infarction. Lateral (V4–V6) and posterior (V7–V9) chest wall leads indicate lateral and posterior myocardial involvement respectively.

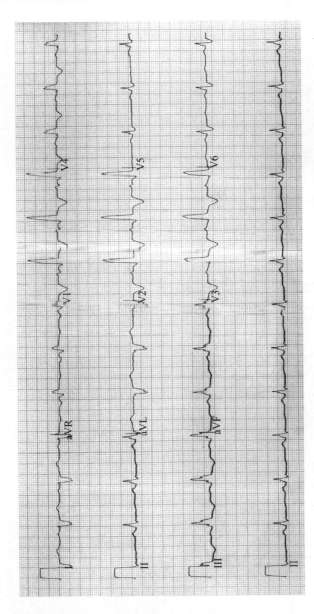

**ECG 26** displays bi-fascicular block: right bundle branch block and left posterior fascicular block (right axis deviation).

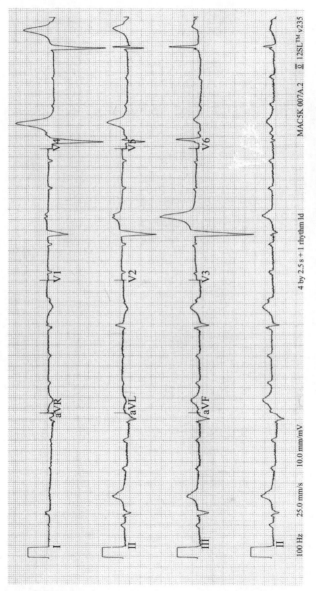

**ECG 27** displays third degree (complete) AV block. It was recorded in an 82-year-old lady who had been admitted with a history of falls and blackouts for the last four weeks, query cause. She was not haemodynamically compromised; her blood pressure was 166/58. She was reviewed by the cardiologist; she remained on an ECG monitor and a permanent pacemaker was arranged. It is important to note the characteristics of the ventricular escape rhythm (see chapter 7).

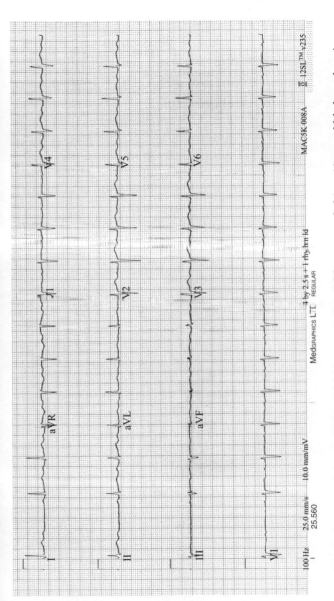

ECG 28 displays second degree AV block Mobitz type 2. This ECG was recorded in a 44-year-old lady undergoing an adenosine street test (Myoview). One minute following the start of the adenosine infusion, the patient developed first degree AV block (prolonged PR interval) and then second degree AV block Mobitz type 2. She was feeling lightheaded. The adenosine infusion was immediately stopped and discontinued. She reverted back to sinus rhythm within two minutes. In this case the AV conduction disturbances were caused by the adenosine.

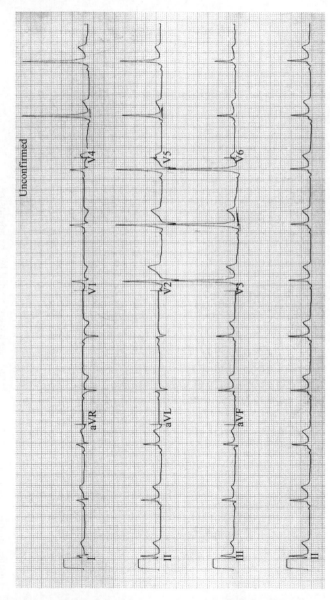

ECG 29 displays *Wolff-Parkinson-White syndrome type A*: left-sided pathway resulting in a predominant R wave. In lead V1, note the short PR interval and delta wave indicating pre-excitation of the ventricles.

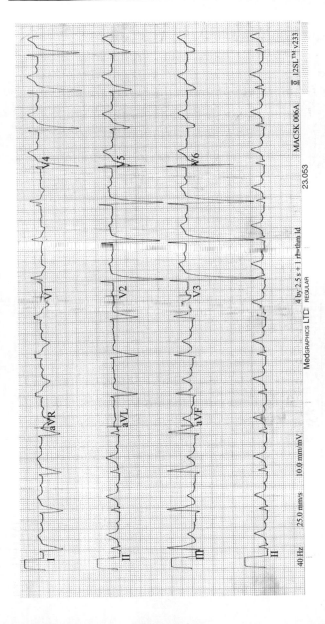

**ECG 30** displays hyper-acute inferior myocardial infarction peaked T waves in II, III and aVF). There is also tri-fascicular block: right bundle branch block, left posterior fascicle block and first degree AV block with a prolonged PR interval).

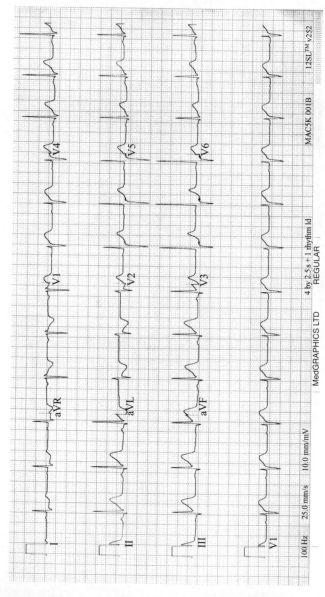

**ECG 31** displays hyperacute inferior ST elevation myocardial infarction. Reciprocal changes can be seen in the lateral leads (I and aVL).

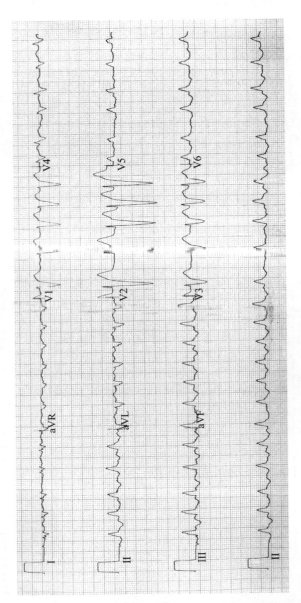

**ECG 32** displays atrial fibrillation with a fast ventricular rate with aberrant conduction.

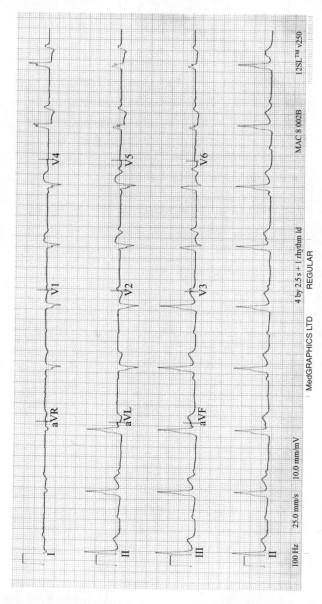

ECG 33 displays third degree AV block. There is complete AV dissociation.

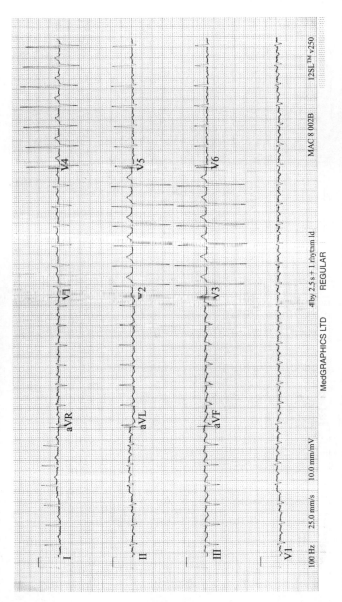

**ECG 34** displays junctional tachycardia. This patient was complaining of chest tightness: ischaemic changes (ST depression/T wave changes) are present in the inferolateral leads.

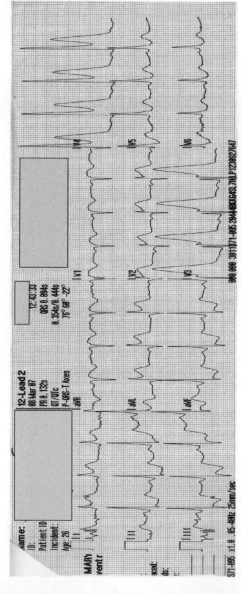

ECG 35 displays acute anterior myocardial infarction. ST elevation is clearly seen in leads 1, aVL, V1–V4; the peaked T waves in V5–V6 suggest that ST elevation will develop in these leads as well. Note the reciprocal changes in the inferior leads (ECG recorded in the pre-hospital setting and reproduced with kind permission from Mark Whitbread, London Ambulance Service).

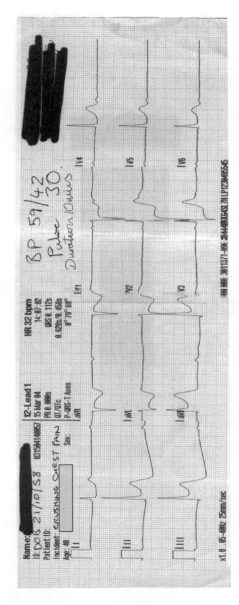

**ECG 36** displays acute inferior/posterior myocardial infarction. ST elevation is clearly seen in leads II, III and aVF. The patient was complaining of central crushing chest pain; his blood pressure was 59/42 and his pulse was 30/min. The ECG shows third degree AV block with a slow ventricular response (30/min) (ECG recorded in the pre-hospital setting and reproduced with kind permission from Mark Whitbread, London Ambulance Service).

# Index

accelerated idioventricular rhythm, 124, 126
definition, 124
causes, 124
effects on the patient, 126
identifying ECG features, 126
treatment, 126
action potential, 2, 3, 4
agonal rhythm, 164
definition, 164–5
causes, 165
ECG examples, 166
effects on the patient, 165
identifying ECG features, 165
treatment, 165
ambulatory cardiac monitoring, 29–31
anterior fascicle, 6
asystole, 159–61
definition, 159
causes, 159
ECG examples, 160
effects on the patient, 161
identifying ECG features, 159, 161
treatment, 161
atrial ectopic beats, 72–7
definition, 72
causes, 73
ECG examples, 76
effects on the patient, 74
identifying ECG features, 73–4
treatment, 74
atrial fibrillation, 87–93
definition, 87–8
causes, 87
ECG examples, 91–2, 263, 268, 281
effects on the patient, 88–9

identifying ECG features, 88
treatment, 89, 227–8
atrial flutter, 80–6
definition, 80
causes, 80
ECG examples, 83, 85–6, 253–4, 271
effects on the patient, 81
identifying ECG features, 81–2
treatment, 81
atrial kick, 72, 88
atrial tachycardia, 77–80
definition, 77
causes, 77
ECG examples, 78, 252, 252
effects on the patient, 79
identifying ECG features, 78–9
treatment, 79
atropine, 7
automaticity, 2, 40–1
autonomic nervous system, 7
AV block, 43
AV dissociation, 189, 256
AV node, 5–7, 13
AV junction, 4–6
AV junctional beats, 96–8
definition, 96
causes, 97
ECG examples, 100
effects on the patient, 97
identifying ECG features, 97
treatment, 98
AV junctional escape beats, 98
definition, 98
causes, 98
ECG examples, 100
effects on the patient, 99

identifying ECG features, 99
treatment, 99
AV junctional escape rhythm, 101–4
    definition, 101
    causes, 101
    ECG examples, 103, 106
    effects on the patient, 102
    identifying ECG features, 101–2
    treatment, 102
AV junctional tachycardia, 104–111
    definition, 104–5
    causes, 105
    ECG examples, 106, 108, 110–111,
        250, 255, 258, 267, 283
    effects on the patient, 105
    identifying ECG features, 105
    treatment, 105
axis deviation, 191, 210

Bachman's bundle, 5
bifascicular bock, 210–13, 275
bradycardia, management of, 222,
    224–5
broad complex tachycardia, irregular,
    treatment of, 223, 228–9
broad complex tachycardia, regular,
    treatment of, 223, 228
bundle of His, 4, 6, 13

calibration, of ECG, 177
capture beat, 127
cardiac arrhythmia, definition of, 40
cardiac arrhythmias, 40–50
    classification of, 43–4
    ECG interpretation of, 44–9
    mechanisms of, 40–3
cardiac monitor, features of, 17–18
complete AV block – see third degree
    AV block
conduction system, 1, 4
coronary artery, 5
coronary care units, history of, 12

depolarisation, 1, 2, 3, 13

EASI 12 lead ECG monitoring, 23–5
ECG, invention of, 11

ECG, relation to cardiac contraction,
    12–13
ECG electrodes, 18, 20, 27–8
ECG gain, 18–19
ECG monitoring, 10–40
    indications for, 13, 15–17
    infection control, 29
    problems associated with, 31–5
    procedure to establish, 25–9,
ECG waveform, configuration of, 178–9
ectopic, definition of, 72
Einthoven's triangle, 177
Einthoven, Willem, 11
electrical axis, 189–191
electrocardiogram, 10
electrocardiography, 10
exercise stress testing, 35–6
external pacing, 238–41
    advantages, 239
    cautions, 240
    indications, 238–9
    percussion pacing, 240
    procedure, 239–40

first degree AV block, 135
    definition, 135–6
    causes, 136
    ECG examples, 138, 264
    effects on the patient, 136
    identifying ECG features, 136
    treatment, 136
fusion beat, 127

hypokalaemia, 260

idioventricular rhythm, 4, 123
    definition, 123
    causes, 123
    ECG example, 125
    effects on the patient, 123
    identifying ECG features, 123
    treatment, 123–4
implantable cardioverter defibrillator,
    237–8

left anterior fascicular block, 191, 210
left axis deviation, 191, 210

left bundle branch, 6, 191, 205, 208–9
left posterior fascicular block, 191, 210
left ventricular hypertrophy, 259

Mason-Likar 12 lead ECG system, 22–3
MCL1, 25
mid-septal fascicle, 6
myocardial infarction, ECG changes,
    191–7
    Q waves, 193–5, 252
    reciprocal changes, 195
    ST segment changes, 192–4
    T wave changes, 192–4
myocardial infarction
    anterolateral, 194, 197, 251, 269
    anteroseptal, 194, 197, 201–2, 262,
        284
    inferior, 194, 196–9, 251, 252, 268,
        273, 274, 279, 280, 285
    lateral, 194, 197, 251, 274
    posterior, 195, 197, 200, 251, 268, 274,
        285
myocardial ischaemia, 15, 197, 203–7,
    270, 271, 283

narrow complex tachycardia, irregular,
    treatment of, 222, 227–8
narrow complex tachycardia, regular,
    treatment of, 222, 226–7
nodal artery, 5

P waves, 11–12, 183–4
pacemaker, permanent, 265
parasympathetic nervous system, 7
peri-arrest arrhythmias, 220–241
    algorithms, use of, 221
    adverse signs, associated with, 221–4
posterior fascicle, 6
PQRST, 11
PR interval, 13, 184–5
pulseless electrical activity, 164
    definition, 164
    causes, 164
    effects on the patient, 164
    identifying ECG features, 164
    treatment, 164
Purkinje fibres, 4, 7, 13,

Q waves, 187, 193, 195, 197
QRS complex, 186–7
QRS rate, 185
QRS rhythm, 185
QT interval, 188–9
QT interval, prolongation of, 13, 16

record keeping, 243–5
    audit of, 246
    common deficiencies of, 244
    importance of, 243–4
    legal issues, 246–8
    principles of, 244–5
repolarisation, 1, 2, 3, 13
resting potential, 2
right axis deviation, 191, 210
right bundle branch block, 191, 208,
    210–211, 213
right ventricular myocardial infarction,
    194

SA node 1, 4, 5, 7, 13
SA block, 64
    definition, 64
    causes, 65
    ECG examples, 66
    effects on the patient, 65
    identifying ECG features, 65
    treatment, 65
second degree AV block Mobitz type
    1, 137–44
    definition, 137, 139
    causes, 139
    ECG examples, 141, 143
    effects on the patient, 140
    identifying ECG features, 139–140
    treatment, 140
second degree AV block Mobitz type
    2, 144–7
    definition, 144
    causes, 144
    ECG examples, 143, 146, 277
    effects on the patient, 145
    identifying ECG features, 144
    treatment, 145
sick sinus syndrome, 68–9
    definition, 68

causes, 68–9
ECG examples, 69
effects on the patient, 69
identifying ECG features, 69
treatment, 69
sinus arrest, 67
definition, 67
causes, 67
ECG examples, 69
effects on the patient, 67–8
identifying ECG features, 67
treatment, 68
sinus arrhythmia, 61
definition, 61
causes, 61
ECG examples, 62, 66, 272
effects on the patient, 63
identifying ECG features, 61
treatment, 63
sinus bradycardia, 55
definition, 55–8
causes, 57
ECG examples, 56, 60
effects on the patient, 57–9
identifying ECG features, 56
treatment, 58
sinus node (see SA node)
sinus rhythm, 13–14
sinus tachycardia, 50–5
definition, 50
causes, 51
ECG examples, 54
effects on the patient, 51–2
identifying ECG features, 51
treatment, 52
ST segment, 188
ST segment depression, 203–5, 250
ST segment elevation, 192–3, 195,
251
sympathetic nervous system, 7
synchronised electrical cardioversion,
229–37
procedure, large adhesive pads,
236–7
procedure, paddles, 234–6
reducing transthoracic impedance,
229–232

safety issues, 232–3
synchronisation with R wave, 233–4

T waves, 11, 13, 188, 192–3, 197, 205
T wave inversion, 203, 206–7
tachycardia, management of, 223,
225–9
telemetry, 29
third degree AV block, 147–53
definition, 147
causes, 147–8
ECG examples, 150, 152, 276, 282,
285
effects on the patient, 149
identifying ECG features, 148–9
treatment, 149
Torsades de pointes, 131–3
definition, 131
causes, 131
ECG example, 133
effects on the patient, 132
identifying ECG features, 131–2
treatment, 132
Trifascicular block, 212, 279
twelve lead ECG, 245–6
twelve lead ECG, interpretation of,
182–218
twelve lead ECG, recording of, 169–180
alternative chest lead placements,
174
calibration, 176
chest leads, position of, 174
indications, 169–170
labelling, 175
procedure, 170–4
posterior, 174
right sided, 174
standardisation of, 175–6
what it records, 176–180

U wave, 11, 189, 260

vagal manoeuvres, 226–7
vagus nerve, 7
ventricular arrhythmias, causes of, 114
ventricular ectopics, 115–121
definition, 115

causes, 115
ECG examples, 118, 120
effects on the patient, 116
identifying ECG features, 116
treatment, 116–7
ventricular escape beats, 121
definition, 121–2
causes, 121
effects on the patient, 122
identifying ECG features, 122
treatment, 122
ventricular fibrillation, 155–9
definition, 156
causes, 156
ECG example, 160
effects on the patient, 157
identifying ECG features, 157
treatment, 157–8
ventricular standstill, 161–3
definition, 161
causes, 161–2
ECG examples, 163
effects on the patient, 162

identifying ECG features, 162
treatment, 162
ventricular tachycardia, 126–31
definition, 126–7
causes, 126–7
ECG examples, 130, 256, 257, 260, 266,
effects on the patient, 128
identifying ECG features, 127–8
treatment, 128

Waller, Augustus, 11
wandering atrial pacemaker, 64
definition, 64
causes, 64
effects on the patient, 64
identifying ECG features, 64
treatment, 64
Wenckeback phenomenon – see
second degree AV block Mobitz
type 1
Wolff-Parkinson-White syndrome, 48,
212, 213–7, 278